BURNT HILLS
VETERINARY TAILS

The life, adventures and legacy of
Stan "Doc" and Shirley Garrison

Written by
Penny Heritage

As told by
S.E. Garrison, D.V.M.

BURNT HILLS
VETERINARY TAILS

The life, adventures and legacy of
Stan "Doc" and Shirley Garrison

Written by
Penny Heritage

As told by
S.E. Garrison, D.V.M.

Published by:
Heritage Farm Publishing
493 Charlton Road
Ballston Spa, NY 12020-3203
www.heritagefarmpublishing.com
e-mail: penny@heritagefarmpublishing.com

International Standard Book Number: 0-9771682-0-4

Library of Congress Control Number: 2005933231

First Edition
Printed in the United States of America

To our daughters
Diane, Linda & Laurel

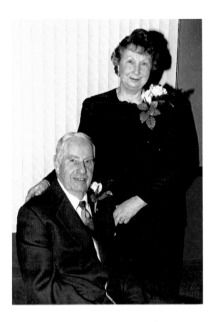

and to Shirley with love from Stan

I have been asked many times "What is the greatest thing you have ever done in your life?" The answer has always been "Marrying Shirley." I thank God and Shirley's parents for bringing this beautiful woman into the world and into my life—she is my constant strength and inspiration. I have always admired her ability to smile throughout life's ups and downs and her distinction of being smart as well as pretty. She has supported my dream as "clerk of the works" in our professional endeavors while at the same time leading our extended family with love and her strong belief in togetherness. I am truly blessed to have Shirley as my life partner.

CONTENTS

INTRODUCTION
By Patricia Thomson Herr, D.V.M.

My first introduction to Dr. Stanley Garrison came sometime in the early 1950's, after our family had been unsuccessfully trying to reach a veterinarian during a spring lambing time emergency. My father, being a fulltime employee at General Electric Company in Schenectady, was a "gentleman farmer" and had decided to raise some chickens and a small herd of sheep. As a teenager, who wanted nothing more than to own her own horse and grow up to be a veterinarian, living on a farm in West Charlton on the border of Schenectady and Saratoga Counties was almost the perfect world.

But lambing season brought its own problems. In particular, our best Corriedale ewe had lambed and now had a large bloody mass extruding from under her tail. After calling several veterinarians and being told they do not treat sheep or "a sick sheep is a dead sheep," we were fortunate enough to reach the Burnt Hills Veterinary Hospital.

Dr. Stanley Garrison arrived at the barn, examined the sheep in question, and explained that it appeared that the ewe's uterus, because of her straining, had prolapsed—or been pushed outside the body. After being told that I wanted to be a veterinarian (like most every other horse-crazy teenager), he suggested I help with the procedure to replace the organ.

The ailing sheep was placed upside down in a nearby wheelbarrow and Dr. Garrison skillfully went to work. Further examination proved that a uterine tumor was a complicating cause. Doubtful that the procedure would be successful, this talented man went ahead with the surgery. When he completed removing this large bleeding mass he threw it to me saying something like, "Here, catch this if you want to be a veterinarian."

I did, and I believe I surprised Dr. Garrison, who continued to explain what he was doing and why and what we needed to do for aftercare. The sheep survived, went on to lamb again the following year, and I became an admirer of Dr. Stanley Garrison and even more convinced that I would become a veterinarian.

Dr. Garrison played an important role in my developing veterinary interests. He invited me to travel along on large animal calls to neighboring farms, allowed me to watch surgeries and treatments at the Burnt Hills Veterinary Hospital and even hired me to work during my summer vacations. What wonderful memories I have of working with Rachel, getting to know Shirley and the girls, and just being a part of that extended family.

When I got a poor grade in my Junior year large animal surgery course, Stan encouraged me to work harder and do better. He was always willing to share his knowledge and be supportive in any way he could.

After marriage to another veterinary student, Donald Herr, we came back to the Capital District and lived for a year at the Burnt Hills Veterinary Hospital, while my husband worked for Stan and I worked for a practice in Glens Falls.

Again, Don and I were benefactors of support from the whole Garrison family. We, as two new graduates, learned the ways of the veterinary profession. Stan Garrison continued to be then, and is even to this day, the finest mentor one could have. He has set an example as an outstanding man in his profession, a fine and loving husband and father, a farmer at heart, and a leader in his community. I know I am only one of many who can speak to the special person Stan is to his family, friends, and community.

Patricia Thomson Herr, D.V.M., was born in Schenectady N.Y., and graduated from the New York State College of Veterinary Medicine at Cornell University in 1960. Along with her husband, Donald Herr, D.V.M., she built and opened the Manheim Pike Veterinary Hospital in 1964. The couple practiced veterinary medicine and raised their three children, Roger, Martha, and Elizabeth in Lancaster, PA. Dr. Herr became the first woman President of the Pennsylvania Veterinary Medical Association in 1989. She chaired the Association's Legislative Committee for many years, and has been a member of the Pennsylvania State Board of Veterinary Medicine for the past six years. The Herr's sold their practice in 2002 and continue to reside in Lancaster.

THE BEGINNING

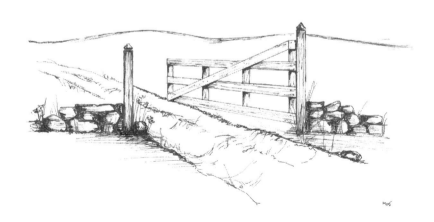

1950
COLLEGE OF VETERINARY MEDICINE
AT CORNELL
ITHACA, NY

During one of our final classes, Dr. Robert McClellan addressed the graduating seniors at the request of the dean. McClellan was a successful D.V.M. from Buffalo, and came to give us some perspective on practicing in the real world. "This post-war class of 1950 is most fortunate," he began, "to have gone through veterinary college with more government funding and the finest equipment to date." In other words, we had the best education—and we shouldn't waste it!

Toward the end of his talk he scanned the room and said, "I suspect someone here is going to go back to his home town to practice." I was sitting in the front row, and was the only one to raise my hand. Dr. McClellan asked to see me after class.

When my classmates had gone, we discussed my future plan to open a veterinary hospital in Burnt Hills. "I didn't mean to say you shouldn't go home, but just think about how difficult that might be. In such a small place, is there enough business to start a practice and keep it going? They'll still think of you as a kid in the town where you grew up..."

I suppose Burnt Hills was a small town when I was a boy, but there was no doubt in my mind—I was going home.

To me, it seemed only logical to return home to start my career. By the time I graduated from veterinary college I was married, with two daughters, and for the past twelve years had been steadily paying the mortgage on our farm. All I wanted to do was to return to Burnt Hills—named for the Mohawk Indians' practice of burning the hills, stimulating new growth on the land—where I had grown up, to raise my own family and build a practice. Somehow I just knew that this wonderful little community in the town of Ballston in Saratoga County would be just the place where we could all flourish.

I can't help but think about a poem that my wife Shirley wrote to me in a Christmas card in 1939, nearly three years before we were married, and ten years before I would even graduate from Cornell. She wrote:

> To the future Dr. Garrison—
> If within your heart you know
> That someday you'll succeed,
> Then no matter how great your dream,
> Or no matter how hard the road,
> You'll always reach the gate
> That opens to your dream.

Looking back on my 87 years, her words seem so appropriate here—my life has been just like a series of gates and paths. When one gate closed and a path ended, it seemed that a special person always opened another gate, guiding me to a different path. This story follows those paths of my childhood on the farm, how I came to practice Veterinary Medicine, and of course, the adventures our own family shared throughout 34 years in practice with the people and animals in this community.

It's been said that if you don't know where you are from, it's hard to know who you are—I guess I have to start my story with my Garrison ancestors' homecomings, including my father's roundabout journey which ended in Burnt Hills.

My great-grandfather, David C. Garrison, was born in 1802 in the town of Galway, Saratoga County, New York. He married Cynthia Wood from the neighboring town of Milton in 1831, and together they had eight children. At some point their family moved to Central New York, but in 1858 at the age of 56, David returned to Saratoga County along with his wife Cynthia, and their youngest son, Charles. They settled on a farm on Goode Road in the town of Milton. Charles was 21 and single then and helped his parents to work the 125-acre farmstead.

Three years later, in 1861, Charles married a young woman who lived just down the road, named Hephzibah Chamberlain. By the time my father was born in 1864, there were already three generations of Garrisons living at the family farm on Goode Road: my great-grandparents David and Cynthia, my grandparents Charles and Hephzibah, and my father David Crosby Garrison.

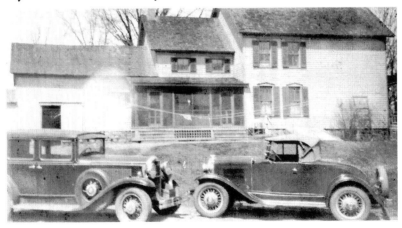

Garrison Homestead at 953 Goode Road, circa 1930

My father was the first child born to Charles and Hephzibah. In 1869, at the age of five, he was joined by a brother, Alden. Sadly, Alden only lived a year before becoming the first family member to be buried in the Garrison cemetery

(South Milton Cemetery) just south of the farm. I never learned the cause, but early childhood deaths were more common at that time. After Alden died, my grandparents decided to head west to the young and growing town of Humboldt, Kansas. Humboldt promised rich, affordable land and a mild climate. It probably seemed easier to farm there than in New York, and attractive for making a fresh start.

For five years they farmed in Humboldt, and in 1875, my father's sister, Ella, was born. All too soon after the joy of their new baby girl, tragedy struck the following spring when Hephzibah died of pneumonia. My father was only 12 years old at the time of his mother's death, and with his father and baby sister, returned home to Milton on the train to bury Hephzibah in the Garrison family cemetery.

Three years passed, and in 1879 my grandfather remarried and my father had a new step-mother, Eva Englehart. Over the next ten years the Garrison family would grow with the arrival of my father's four half-brothers: Albert (Bert) in 1880, Charles Leonard (Len) in 1888, and the twins Alfred and Arthur in 1889.

By the time the twins were born my father was already in his twenties and felt the need to branch out on his own. He traveled the country doing all kinds of different things, hoping to discover just what he wanted to do. He spent some time back in Kansas taking agricultural courses at the university, and even visited his uncles and cousins in Minnesota while in the Midwest.

In 1893 he entered a bicycle relay race from Boston to New York continuing all the way to Chicago. It was at a rest-stop in the race in East Greenbush, New York, at a corn husking bee of all things, that he met my mother Katherine "Kate" Goodman. Her parents, John and Mary Dine Goodman had come to America with a group of families when they were young. John, a veteran of the Civil War, came from Alsace-Lorraine, and Mary had been born in Germany.

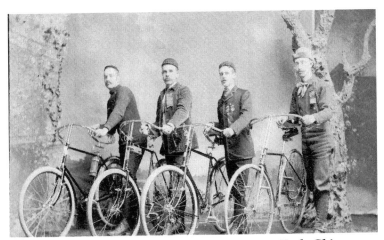

**Ballston Riders in The Great Boston-New York-Chicago
Relay Bicycle Race, April 30th-May 4th, 1893
(David C. Garrison- 2nd from left)**

They'd settled in the East Greenbush area and raised six kids in addition to Kate: Matthew, Joseph, Albert, John, Anna, and Tillie. When the bicycle race ended in Chicago, my father stuck around. That's where he got interested in buying and selling livestock at the stockyards. He'd always thought about going into farming but never had the money.

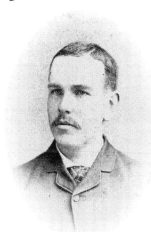

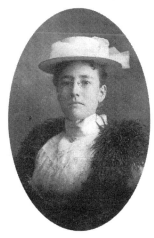

David C. & Katherine E. Garrison

I don't know when my father moved back to New York, or much about their courtship, but in 1898 my parents, David and Katherine Garrison, were married at the First Baptist Church in Amsterdam, New York. I have their pretty little marriage certificate where my mother's name appears as "Kittie". I always thought that it was unusual to use a nickname on such a formal document. My father had a good job at the Amsterdam Meat Packing Company by that time, so he and my mother decided to stay in the area and start a family. My brother Melvin was born in 1900, joined by my sister Edith in 1901 and Anna Mae in 1904.

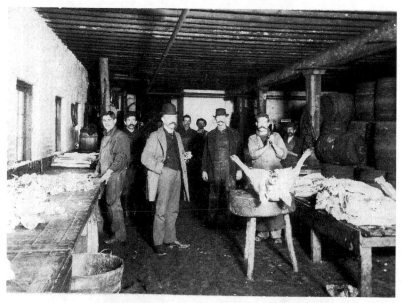

Amsterdam Packing Company 1909
(David C. Garrison, 3rd from left)

After ten years in the meat packing business, my dad decided that he wanted to get back to farming more than ever. Without much to invest, he bought a small farm on Peaceable Street and Birchton Road in the town of Galway, which was quite close to my Aunt Ella Armer's farm. That was where my sister Laura was born in 1909. After only a year, my dad realized that the farm wasn't the right place for him. My brother Melvin recalled plowing the fields at the Birchton farm and picking more stones than potatoes on that piece of ground!

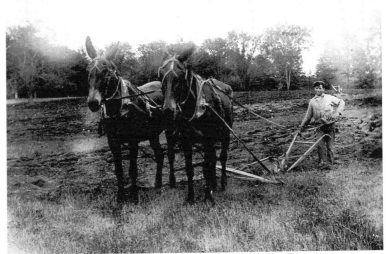

Melvin & mules plowing at Birchton Farm

Dad sold the farm in Birchton and bought a house on Laurel Avenue in Schenectady. He worked fixing up houses in the city, saving his money until he could find the right farm. The following year my Uncle Bert told him about a farm he'd heard was for sale.

It was in 1911 that my parents made their final move to the farm on Goode Street in Burnt Hills. Ironically, this farm was just six miles south of the place where my father had been born. At the turn of the century, the thirty square mile town of Ballston (where Burnt Hills is located) had a population of just 2,000.

My dad purchased the Goode Street farm from a man named Charles Cady VanVorst. The property had a beautiful house set back off the road that had been built in 1869 as well as several outbuildings. It really was a picture—still is today! The large hip-roof barn (120' x 30') assembled with wooden pegs, had been added in 1900 by two local carpenters and a group of volunteers. It had been one of the last barn raisings in the area. The women of the Methodist Church even fed all of the folks who came out to help. While the barn had been set up for an expanded herd of 40 cows, it never housed Mr. VanVorst's small milking herd, which still fit in the old barn. VanVorst was much more of

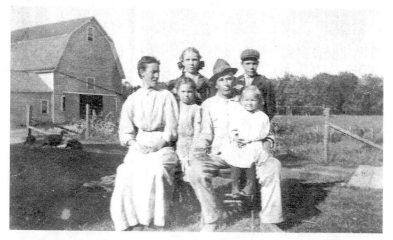

David C. Garrison Family at Goode Street Farm, 1911

an entrepreneur than a farmer, buying and wholesaling grain, storing it in big steel bins to keep the mice out. After my father bought the farm an auction was held to sell off the stock and farming implements. A flier for the auction advertised four horses and a colt, eleven cows and a bull, a gobbler and turkeys, and some small equipment and tools—sums over ten dollars payable to the Union National Bank of Schenectady.

The move to Goode Street proved to be a good one. I consider myself fortunate to have had my folks pick such a fine place for us to live and make our home. My sister Mabel was born there in 1915 and I came along three years later.

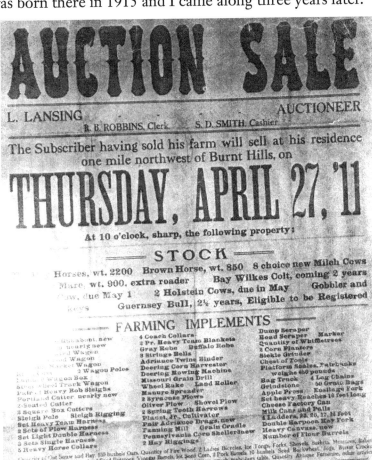

Charles C. Van Vorst Farm Auction, 1911
Announcement printed in Ballston Spa Daily Journal

I was born at home on March 15th in 1918... and that's not yesterday! It wasn't a big deal at the time to be born at home, in fact, most people were, and I was the tip of the litter. As my mother was getting ready to bring her sixth child into the world, she calmly talked to Dad at the breakfast table that morning. Dad went to see Dr. Cotton—the only doctor in the area—when he went to deliver the milk down to Burnt Hills. Dr. Cotton promised to come right up to the farm after he finished his office hours. It must've been one heck of a snowy day because Dr. Cotton's one-horse cutter got stuck in the drifts by McKnight's place, about a mile down the road. He managed to shovel his sleigh out but had to come back the next day. No one was too worried that he didn't make it though, because my sisters were there to help with the delivery. It worked out well for me in the end—for several years we celebrated my birthday over two days! My dad was tickled to have another boy after four girls in a row, and my mother said he rolled me over several times to make sure I had all the essentials. By the time I was born, Dad was 55 years old, and my mother was 12 years younger.

The year I was born turned out to be pretty eventful— my mother always talked about how many things happened in 1918. My dad bought a Model-T Depot Hack for about $700 that year to celebrate the arrival of a son, and in November, my parents bundled me up, rolled the side curtains down, and took me to Schenectady for the Armistice Day parade. There wasn't any room for my brother or sisters because there were two butchered pigs in the back of the truck to deliver to Nicholaus' Restaurant.

At a young age, I became aware that my dad was really a jack-of-all-trades. He made harnesses, whippletrees, and eveners to hitch the horses, and even resoled our shoes. He seemed to be able to do everything right there on his workbench. My dad would come in from the barn at noon most days, have a meal, and then take a short nap. He often said everybody should take a nap at noon—even the dog.

On top of being versatile with his work, he was an intelligent man, and could read exceptionally fast. All the old guys down at the little barbershop in Burnt Hills would ask him, "Dave, what's new in current events?" and he could spell it right out for them. Most of the men went to Bayliss' barbershop just to get a shave and talk. The barbershop was something that really should have been saved in Burnt Hills because it was a special gathering place. It was a small, square building across the road from Dr. Cotton's, just north of the pole that flew the flag in Burnt Hills where Kingsley Road meets Lakehill Road. At that time it was the center of Burnt Hills, and the roads in each direction were called East, West, North, and South Street. This was all before Route 50 went through.

Dad had a wide range of interests. When he traveled around the country as a young fellow, he became a bit interested in theater and opera. We couldn't imagine such a thing… running a farm and being interested in theater! When some of our relatives from the Midwest visited us they brought Dad along with them to the opera in New York City. It never sounded like anything that us kids would like. My mother didn't think too much of it either.

My mother was a practical nurse and worked for Dr. Cotton. When they needed her, patients would ring a little bell to get her attention. We still have that bell! After someone had a baby, she would often spend two to three days at the home caring for the family and helping out. A lot of times she wound up staying for other situations as well.

When Dr. Cotton didn't need her services my mother was more than busy around the farm. She was great at making clothes, a wonderful cook, and responsible for all of the housekeeping, gardening, and canning. She taught us kids to help with things as we got older, but did most of the day-to-day work necessary to keep our family going. She drove the horses, but never a car. When they were old enough, the girls

18

took her wherever she wanted to go. I can still see her carrying a cast iron teakettle full of hot water to the barn to wash up the milking machine; the kettle itself was heavy enough to handle. She was a strong woman in so many ways.

MY SIBLINGS

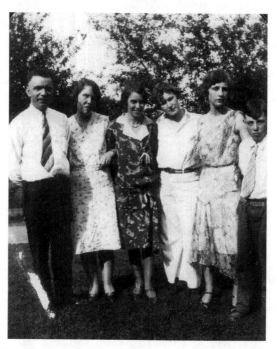

(L-R) Melvin, Edith, Anna Mae, Laura, Mabel, & Stan

I believe that I had the best childhood you could ask for! There were six of us kids—a boy on each end and four girls in the middle.

Melvin was the oldest, and when he was just a boy he trained a bull to pull him around in a little cart. By the time I was born, Melvin was already 18 years old. He was very clever with machinery, especially gasoline engines and motorcycles. He didn't like the horses, and seemed to get kicked every time he got close to them. My dad made a deal with Melvin, "You take care of the machinery and I'll take care of the horses." And that worked out fine.

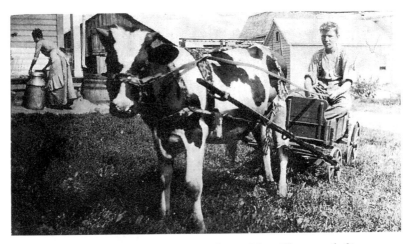

Melvin in his bull cart (Mother with milkcan at left)

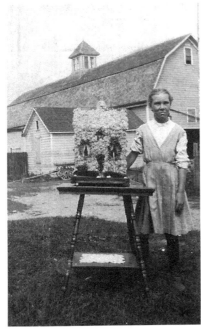

Edith's Straw Flower Clock

My sister Edith came next. She did a lot of things at home, like cooking with my mother, but was also creative and quite handy. She once made a steeple clock out of straw flowers that she took to the Ballston Fair. Melvin hooked up the pendulum inside of it. The clock was decorated with letters and flowers dyed in different colors, and was really quite something. She showed it at the fair and won $40. Some years later, when Charles Lindbergh landed here, my brother suggested making an airplane out of straw flowers, so Edith did!

Anna Mae didn't show as many things at the fair as Edith, but she helped my mother with the cooking and cleaning as well. Since they were older, the girls took care of all of us. Anna Mae got the job of washing the diapers out—she probably would have liked to have burned them! She was a good sport though, and learned to be a real homemaker.

My sister Laura didn't have any interest in cooking. She was the tomboy of the family and took over helping my dad after Melvin was grown and had moved out. I can remember her with a grease rag and a crescent wrench in her back pocket. In 1927, when she was close to finishing high school, Laura and some girls decided to wear slacks to school just for fun. Laura was the leader of the group, and they all got suspended for this. Some of the girls bobbed their hair at that time, and even a few teachers went along with them. When the school board met with my dad to discuss the slacks incident he said, "Well, Laura wears coveralls around home all the time." She always looked good. She'd steam her hair before she went out, and wear a white bib-top and slacks. When they told her she couldn't wear slacks to school, she decided to quit and went to the G.E. and got a good job. She was an innovator and received many cash awards for her ideas. At G.E. she headed up the assembly line with 16-18 girls under her; Laura was a real achiever and a leader among women. In 1929 she bought a brand new Buick which made her really independent. She was one of a kind, all right.

Mabel and I were the only two kids born on Goode Street. My brother and three sisters were older, and by the time we were grown, everyone else had either gotten married or had a job at General Electric. Mabel was my mentor in a lot of ways and we played together as kids. Back then nobody had very much in the way of toys and games, so Mabel and I pretended to be these characters called Lena & John T. Shanty. My mother put together a suitcase with clothes for us to dress up in and we'd go out and put on a show for our neighbors. Mabel and Laura taught me how to dance when I was six or seven years old; they were fun to be around and excellent role models. They both did well in school. When the roads were clogged with snow and the teachers couldn't get home, my sisters brought Miss McChesney and Miss Rice to our house to stay the night. These teachers both wanted Mabel and Laura to go on to college but they didn't. Laura had quit after she got suspended and Mabel decided to get married when she was a senior. None of my sisters or my brother ever finished high school, although I know they were all smarter than I was. Everyone followed their own course as circumstances allowed.

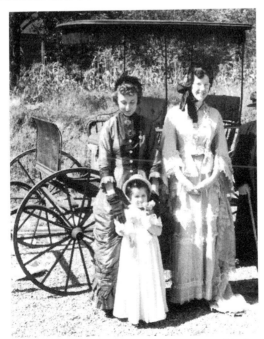

My sister, Mabel Rogers, (left) with Joyce Wolfe (center) and Phyllis Kimbell (right) at the Burnt Hills Methodist Church Lord's Acre Auction in 1950

LIFE ON OUR FARM

There was always a job on the farm for everyone—tailored to their size and ability to do it. I remember the girls taking care of the lamps and lanterns for the barn—they trimmed the wicks and filled them with kerosene. The lanterns were hung four feet from the ceiling so nothing could catch on fire. Like most others, our family was fearful of fire, and extra careful because there was no insurance. My dad wouldn't let anyone smoke around the barn, and we were one of the first farmers around to put lightning rods on the cupola.

My jobs around the farm were little at that time—but so was I! I filled the wood box and got kindling. It wasn't much of a job but pretty important. We always needed to have kindling ready for morning when my dad started the fire about five o'clock. He used to say when I was still quite small, "When you go out to get the cows in the morning, check your shoes—if they're wet from the heavy dew, it probably won't rain, so we'll cut hay." That sounds kind of funny, but there was no electricity or radio in the barn to hear the weather forecast, so it was our own way of telling what we might do that day. My dad also said that if the leaves on the hickory tree were as big as a squirrel's ears, then it was time to plant corn. These are some of the little things I remember as a kid.

Milk was our main source of income on the farm. We had 35 cows and used a Hinman milking machine with a gasoline engine. We didn't do much milking by hand even before electricity came. We got about two dollars a hundredweight (a hundred pounds of milk) at that time, and took the cans to Turpit's store in Burnt Hills (and later to Rankin's Dairy in Scotia) every day. The night's milk had to be chilled down, and the morning's milk was taken as it was. Farmers were required to stay up to date with concrete floors in the milk room and to keep it clean.

My mother would get up at 6:00 every morning to start the oatmeal for breakfast, which was set on the back of the stove overnight—I can still hear that thing popping and popping. Everyone would come in for breakfast at 7:00 like clockwork, with the milking done and the cattle and horses fed. The livestock ate before we ate. That was important. There was a time, three years in a row, when 10 people—six of us kids, my mother and father, grandmother Goodman and our hired man—sat around the long oval table to eat. My granddaughter Darlene is using this table at the home farm where she now lives. On Sundays there were sometimes more than that. My mother was a great cook and my dad was a great provider.

The same woodstove that our oatmeal was cooked on was used for so many things, including heating the soft water from the cistern in a big copper boiler for Monday's wash. I remember my mother making handsoap and my job was to wrap the bars with newspaper and put them out of the way for storage on the steps to the attic, which were steep as a ladder. The stove also heated the kitchen where we spent most of our time in the winter. We went to bed at 9:00 and if the fire went out at night, the reservoir used to freeze over, believe it or not. This doesn't say much for our house's insulation, but ours was still one of the better ones at that time. When it was needed, that reservoir was boiling with water. Melvin once made a pair of hickory skis for Mabel by bending the nose of them in that reservoir. The stove had everything—even a warming oven so if somebody was late for dinner, his meal would be put up top to keep it warm.

Our jobs around the farm changed with the seasons. When it came to wintertime, we had to have at least one pair of horses shod in order to get the ice harvested. My dad, having lived in Amsterdam, knew a lot of people over there. He would drive one team of horses to Amsterdam before

Thanksgiving to have shoes put on. That 30 mile drive had to have been a long and cold one!

We used to think of all the places where we could get ice—sometimes it was off of the creek, sometimes off of someone's pond. Dad finally built a pond on the back part of our farm. We filled our icehouse and even supplied ice to Markham's bakery, Turpit's store, and several other businesses around here. When somebody was cutting ice and fell through, as Melvin did once, they'd have to walk all the way home frozen stiff, and just change clothes before heading back out.

On Christmas Eve we would cut down a tree from our property, put it up in the parlor (which was only heated during that time of the year), and decorate it all in the same day. My mother made cookies and left them by the stairway. We all knew just where to go to help ourselves.

Christmas time always meant that my dad would be butchering. He knew how to cure pork and beef from his days at the packing company in Amsterdam. We had a pork barrel in the cellar to put the hams and the shoulders in, and Dad would tell me to go out to the chicken coop and get two fresh eggs to check the salt concentration of the brine. If the eggs floated, then we knew we had the right specific gravity. After the meat had been in that salt brine for so many days, he hung it in our small smokehouse down by the pond. We used hickory bark and corncobs to smoke the meat. We didn't want a fire; we just wanted to keep it smoking.

The wood ashes from the hickory bark, along with baking soda, made up the toothpaste we used as kids. Since money was so tight everyone was resourceful and used every bit for something.

When springtime came around and the snow melted, we'd see more of our neighbors. George and Cora McKnight lived on Goode Street below us, and Herb and Lela

VanVorst lived across from them. The McKnights had no children—Cora was the town clerk for Ballston and George ran their small farm. We'd pick up their two cans of milk, which were never full as their few cows didn't produce a lot, and take it with ours to Burnt Hills. The VanVorsts were similar to the McKnights with a small operation and not many hands to help, and my dad would send me down to help saw up firewood for them. Neither family had much machinery, and they didn't plant any oats, so there was no combining to do. They didn't fill silo either. They stored the hay from their fields and fed it out over the winter, but every spring they were short, and needed a load or two. I remember one March when we were loading hay from our old steep-roofed barn to take down to McKnight's and my job was to tread the hay down and watch the lines on the horses. The horses were right under the eaves of the roof when the snow let loose. They were so spooked they took off down the lane, and were almost to McKnight's before I could stop them.

When the frost went out of the ground in spring we'd fix fence with our neighbors, the Merchants. All that separated our farm and theirs were four strands of barbed wire, so we'd work together—Steve Merchant, Sr. and his son Albert on one side, and my dad and I on the other. Two of us would put up the wire while the other two fixed the post. We did that early in the spring to keep the cattle on the right side of the fences. If the job lasted through noontime, we had our lunch with us and ate together.

In summertime the grass was green and the cows produced more milk, so the extra milk went to Bischoff's Chocolate Factory in Ballston. We tried not to have a surplus in the summer when the price was low; instead, we tried to have the cows freshen (calve) in September when the price of milk was high.

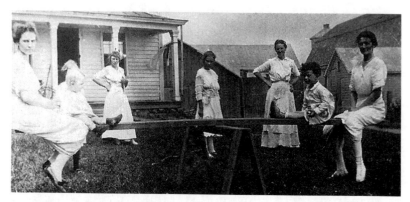

Family group taking turns enjoying a makeshift seesaw
(Edith at left, back and Katherine, my mother,
standing at center right)

Every year on the 4th of July we had a few sparklers and celebrated the end of haying. My dad would say that you should have your haying done by Independence Day, and then plant the buckwheat. When the crop was ready, we sold the buckwheat to Mr. Parkis in Ballston Lake. He had two silos where he stored the grain and made buckwheat pancake flour. In the wintertime the churches would buy the buckwheat flour and put on pancake suppers to raise money. This was a big thing in our area.

We didn't do any butchering in the summer, but if we needed beef, my dad had contacts with some of the big meat suppliers in Schenectady. One supplier named Mr. Wasserman would sell us a quarter of beef, which my mother would have to cut up into pieces, and put in the pressure cooker to can and preserve. I can remember her getting up a couple times in the night to change those big mouth quart jars. There was no refrigeration in those days, so she had to keep canning until the job was done.

Farmers would often contact my dad when they had cattle to sell. He took me on one of these calls to meet a man who had about 22 head of cattle he wanted to sell. We went to look at them, and instead of saying he didn't like the cattle, my dad said to the man, "Henry, I think your cows are bigger than the stalls in my barn—I don't think my stanchions will hold 'em." This was a nice way of letting him down easy.

The summer kitchen on the farmhouse was a busy place. All of the canning of fruits and vegetables got done out there, and everybody showed up in the month of August to help. There was an outhouse about 200 feet away that we used only in the summer. You could tell if someone was in there because the piece of hickory wood that held the door closed would be rotated sideways. Us kids used to spin that wood button, which would upset the person inside. No one wanted to get locked in the outhouse!

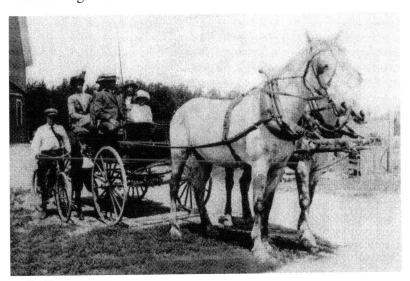

Family in buggy, going to the Burnt Hills Baptist Church

Our drinking water came from a well in front of the house. It wasn't very deep but it provided fine, cold water. Our only refrigeration was an icebox in the kitchen that had a pan beneath it to catch water from the melting ice. We sold our best ice and used the rest ourselves. Sometimes it had been cut close to the dirt and might contain frozen amphibious creatures that hibernated in winter. One summer, when relatives were visiting, somebody forgot to change the pan of water, and a frog and a fish were flopping across the floor!

When we were young kids, Albert Merchant, Dewitt Jenkins, Bud Knight, Lee Hammond and I started a circus. Jenkins had a cow named "Mike" and we made a fence for her out of baling twine. She took it down, wrapping her horns all up in it. We had a horse named Mae, and Lee Hammond had a four-legged chicken. My father made a birdhouse with a sign that said, "Come and see the golden bats," and in it were two little baseball bats. The circus was a penny outfit that didn't last long, but everybody contributed and had fun.

Clarence Knight, who lived on Goode Street, had a large apple orchard. He was my Sunday School teacher and used to pick me up for Sunday school, so I got to know him pretty well. When the Conklingville Dam opened, he took his son Alton ("Bud") and me fishing. We caught some big fish too—they were mostly Pike. When we got back, they dropped me off with my fish at the end of our lane, and I spotted two raccoon babies whose mother had been killed in the road. I brought out a small bucket with some honey left in the bottom, and opened the container up with a pair of tin shears so those two babies could put their heads in there to eat.

I remember visiting my Uncle Len, Aunt Sate Garrison, and my cousins, Roy and Earl at their farm just six miles north on Goode Road where my dad was born. Uncle Len said to my dad, "Why don't you let Stanley come up for a week and see what the farmhouse you lived in was like?" In the morning Uncle Len and my cousins would have the greatest discussions after breakfast about what they were going to do that day—"Should we kill the Barred Rocks or the Rhode Island Reds?" When it was all done, Uncle Len was always the one who made the decision. They were constantly betting just for fun—they would bet a new hat on what the bull weighed before he was butchered, or other things like that.

Summer was also when we went in the Model-T to visit my mother's family in East Greenbush. It was one of the few trips we took to a neighboring county. The ride to visit just for pleasure and change of scenery made it exciting. The East Greenbush area was noted for its gardens and my mother's family grew all kinds of plants and flowers.

The term "changing works" has been all but forgotten today. It meant taking turns, neighbors helping neighbors, when there was a job too big to do alone. Most farms at that time didn't hire outside help, and when it came to threshing the oats, or filling silo, they used to change works. If there was only half a day's work at one farm, and a full day at another, it didn't make any difference—nobody kept track of the time. On a bigger farm like the Rowledge's, which was just west of our farm on Jenkins Road, there was much more to do, but everybody was glad to help. The women would put on a special meal out on the lawn and the men could wash up, eat, and enjoy themselves. It always seemed like the hottest day of the year when we were changing works.

My mother's birthday was near Halloween and she always enjoyed dressing up. It was special for us kids too, because she'd take time and come with us to visit the neighbors' houses for goodies. I remember one Halloween we went to see Buell Hall, who was getting his gun ready to go hunting. I tapped on one of his windows—which I shouldn't have done—and he grabbed his gun and came out. I was scared to death.

Late in the fall, we'd put the potatoes down in the cellar so we'd have them to sell all winter long. In the spring we sold any that were left for seed potatoes. We had the first potato digger in the area—even though we only grew three acres of them. We raised cabbage and carrots too. There was always something to sell as a cash crop, including baby piglets as soon as they were eight weeks old.

As tight as things were, we never felt poor. We didn't have much money, but everybody around was poor. People were losing their homes, farms and cattle. Regardless, I can't remember a time when we didn't have plenty of food to eat—even through the Depression years.

VISITORS

It was very seldom that strangers came to the farm, other than the Rawleigh Man. He came in the spring to sell supplies like Pain King (a mentholated liniment made from wood alcohol), skunk oil (to cure laryngitis), and whatever else he might have. Our place was about 800 feet off the road, and once in a while a butcher would come in to buy a calf. My sister used to scare me with threats that the family would trade me for something.

Our road did become popular after a while. People would come up from Burnt Hills looking for Jenkins Road, which was the next road above us, and they would turn into our lane. My dad ended up putting a sign on the tree at the end that said "Private Road". Mabel and I used to feel kind of important sitting behind that tree waiting for a ride to school.

People who did visit regularly were neighbors who had cattle to breed. There was no artificial breeding in the area at that time, and the cattle would be walked up to the farm and left for the day to be bred. I can remember the book my mother had to record the income—it was one dollar for each cow bred.

THE VETERINARIAN AND OUR ANIMALS

Before veterinarians were common, most farmers treated their own animals when they were sick. The first time Dr. Harry Hansen came from Ballston Spa to the farm, which would have been about 1933, was for a case of Acetonemia. Nobody had heard of that before. We had a Jersey cow out in the pasture by the barn who had wandered over by the woods and was acting drunk, staggering around in circles. It would take her 20 minutes just to get into the barn. After inspecting the cow, Harry said, "Well, it could be Grass Tetany (a magnesium deficiency), but it's probably a sugar problem." So we had to give her two bottles of sugar (an energy supplement with electrolytes). She recovered almost instantly, and I thought it was like a miracle! Dr. Hansen's second trip to our farm was to treat a cow with Milk Fever (hypocalcemia). He came down and only charged three dollars for the call and medicine.

In addition to cows, we had lots of chickens that my mother took care of. We didn't have sheep, but we had pigs—three sows that would have piglets twice a year. The barn was also always full of cats… even some Manx.

We always had a dog—usually a big shepherd, who would sit under the table near me. I couldn't stand fat meat. My father said that's the only way to have flavor, but I couldn't stomach it—so I would cut it off and slide it under the table to the dog. I fed him all the fat meat I couldn't eat. When the dog got so old he couldn't run, my dad half-jokingly said to my mother, "Kate, I don't think we'll get another dog—Stan can outrun any dog we got."

Every horse on the farm was a workhorse; we didn't have ponies, but always had a bunch of mares. My dad always had Belgians. He wouldn't have a stallion or boar hog because they were too dangerous—he said it was bad enough to have a bull.

Anybody who needed a pair of draft horses would come see my dad; he had three teams of mares that delivered foals every year. That was a cash crop. Spring was the happiest time on the farm—the green grass and flowers were coming and the little foals were running around with legs too long for their bodies. Our rural area was beautiful. I just can't remember a time when we didn't have a pasture full of baby foals in April or May. My mother told me that I enjoyed watching the foals even as a tot. When the grass was quite tall, the mares would hide their newborn foals. Edith would take me by the hand and we'd look through the rail fence to try and spot any babies. She'd get me all excited when she shouted, "I see something out there!" I'd run over to my dad, grab ahold of him, and we'd check it out. I'd follow my big sister's example and exclaim in my wee little voice, "I see sumpin'... you see sumpin' too, Pa?" Those foals were an attraction for everybody that came by.

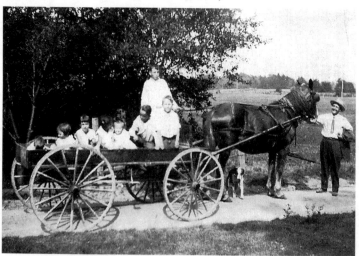

Wagon full of kids, Stan at the reins

It was part of my job as I got a little older to help teach the foals. We would hitch a pair of horses to the bobsleigh with the foals alongside, and train them through the snow. When they became two years old and had been broke to drive, there were plenty of people looking for a team.

Mr. Van Campen, a farmer from Ballston Lake, wanted a team of horses one time. My father had a young pair that had been partially broke, and Mr. Van Campen asked if they had any vices. I guess I knew what a vice was by then because I spoke up and told him that they always jumped up in the manger with their front feet when we watered them. My confession didn't ruin the purchase, but my father took me aside afterward and taught me the finer points of salesmanship.

All of our horses were brought up on sulfur water, and when sawdust fell down through the cracks from the ice-house into the well, the water became pretty briney. The foals just loved it and that was the taste our horses were used to. When we went over to Don Rowledge's farm to do the threshing, we had to take water with us in a milkcan for the horses, otherwise they wouldn't drink. My dad often reluctantly told the story about the time he went to Rowledge's to help put oats in, and Don said to him "Gee it's nice you brought your grandson." Dad was 55 years old when I was born, so he might have been 65 at that time, and I was just 10. You can bet my dad straightened him out on that.

Working with horses was always enjoyable—not a chore or drudgery. Machinery was becoming more available at that time, and could do most of the tasks faster and easier, but my dad loved the horses. One day down at the barbershop somebody asked him, "Dave, why do you still keep horses when you've got tractors?" Dad replied, "I've never seen a tractor replace itself." My brother Melvin was the mechanic and he kept things going on the farm, while my dad spent time with me working with the horses. After all, that was the agreement they had made.

My father was a good horseman, but he'd had an accident driving horses when he was younger, and pulled his shoulder out. He was very careful about it, but Dr. Cotton showed me how to put it back in just in case. I did that for him one day while he lay on the ground in the snow. I had to twist it just right and get it to snap. I remember him going home holding it and walking. "I don't want to ride," he said, "I'll walk."

LOOKING BACK...1923 WAS A BIG YEAR

When I was five years old my father handed me our 1923 license plate that had come in the mail. He said, "You're old enough now, you can fasten that plate onto the back of the Model-T." It went on the back because the cars had a crank start—the plate couldn't have gone on the front, or you'd lose your hand. We kept that Model-T for a long, long time and I still have that license plate today.

At the end of that summer of '23, three big things all happened in one week. The first was that I got my first haircut at Dave Bayliss' barbershop. Before we'd left the house my mother told Dad, "Here's a bag for you to bring some of those curls back." I felt kind of foolish in the barbershop getting my hair cut with all the men in there. They had to put a board on top of the barber chair for me to sit high enough, and I could see everybody watching me.

The second big event to occur was getting ready to go to the Ballston Fair. We didn't go very many places, but the county fair was only once a year for a few days in August, and was really something. We used to have a picnic lunch with the Garrisons and the Armers up at the fair in the back field under a tree. Everybody brought a big spread and it was a fun thing to do. Before we left for the fair, my mother told me, "Go out to the hen house and gather the eggs—they'll get too warm if we leave them in there all day." I had a small basket, but it wouldn't hold all the eggs, so I stuck one in each front pocket to take to the house. The fair was a special occasion and I wore little linen shorts, which I never would have worn on the farm. I remember our Model-T having trouble going up the fairground hill (it didn't have a fuel pump on the gas line—just gravity feed) so Dad turned it around, and backed up the hill. When I saw the ferriswheel, I was so excited that I slapped my thighs. Turns out those eggs were still in my pockets and the sticky mess slid all the way down to my ankles before we had even gotten to the fair. I'll never forget it. I had a hard time convincing my mother not to take me back home.

The day after we went to the fair I started school—the third big event in my life at the time. In the fall, we always made a trip to Montgomery Wards in Latham just before cold weather came. After harvesting we had the time and money from the crops to buy the few things we needed.

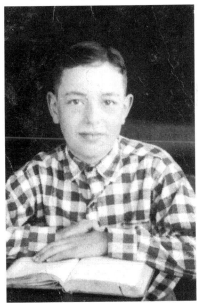

Stan "cracking the books" during his early school days

Mabel and I went to a small, one-room schoolhouse on Scotchbush Road, on the backside of our farm—just about a mile or so away. Stanley Liebert lived across the road from the school, and we started first grade together. I remember that we held hands on that first day because we were afraid to go to school to begin with, and secondly, because our teacher's name was Miss Tygert. We couldn't get over that—the tiger name scared us to death. By the middle of January she got married to George Hunter, so we felt better that George Hunter got ahold of her.

The tiny schoolhouse was a nice place to get an education, with a lot of personal attention, and eight grades all together. In the winter, my dad took us to school through the fields with the horse and sleigh on his way to deliver the milk. The school had a potbelly woodstove with a big agate kettle on top, and that's where the drinking water went. We got our water from a pipe that was filled by a water-activated ram down in the creek and flowed uphill to a concrete tank. Several trout floated around in the tank, and the cows came over and drank out of it. In the spring and fall, it was no problem walking that short distance to the schoolhouse. This was a great place to start school for my first year. I only went there for one year, and Mabel went for three.

The next year, we went to the BH-BL school across from Frank Gardner's farm in Ballston Lake. This school was built on Lakehill Road in 1916, and was called the Burnt Hills-Ballston Lake School of Agriculture and Homemaking. The first graduating class of 1920 only had two people. It was 1924 when I went there for second grade, and our school was the second consolidated district in the state—unbelievable for a small little area like ours. We were transported to school by Merchant's truck, which was normally used to deliver apples and potatoes. They just slid in some seats, pulled the side curtains down, and that's how we went to school. I remember Dave Palmer stopping one morning to pick me up and having a potato roll out by my feet. I handed it back, and he put it on the dash where it stayed for the longest time.

One winter, while driving us to the Christmas pageant at school in the Model-T, my dad got stuck on Lakehill Road. Luckily, some boys from the farm school came along and helped push him out.

Our school had a fire in 1930 when I was in 7th grade and we all were dispersed to various churches and buildings in the community. I was sent to the Odd Fellows Hall for school, and my job was to bring water over for our class from the Methodist Church. That year our teacher, Miss Murray, who belonged to the teachers association, brought back pencils from Ticonderoga for everyone. Miss Murray and the rest of the teachers made do with their makeshift classrooms, and we were all back in the big school the next year when it was rebuilt.

ELECTRICITY & THE TELEPHONE

In 1927 electricity came to our farm. It had been at Knight's to the north of us and down Goode Street to the poultry farm, but had not come all the way to our farm. The electric company needed power poles, and my dad sold them over 50 chestnut poles at $50 apiece. The blight had come through earlier and killed the chestnut trees. This was an unexpected windfall, and amounted to a lot of money at that time. When my dad sold the poles he asked my mother, "Kate, what would you like for the house?" Up until then we never bought many things for the house—everything went to the barn, but my mother never complained. She said she would like a kitchen cabinet with lots of drawers. Barney's had a special cabinet with an agate tray, and silverware drawer, a flour bin and sifter on one side, and a sugar bin on the other. This kitchen cabinet is still in the family. My granddaughter Amy has it in her home.

When electricity went in, the telephone accompanied it, and it was just like another world. We had instant communication with our neighbors, friends and relatives without having to travel and speak face to face. Along with electricity came brighter lighting, and soon new appliances that introduced a different means to cook, wash, iron, and do other everyday chores. Since electricity was a new addition to homes, the wiring was exposed and not hidden inside the walls. My father was both skeptical and a little bit fearful and wanted the best wiring for safety.

TB

Around 1928, cattle were being tested for bovine tuberculosis. The first test was a pill that was put in the corner of the cow's eye—if it clouded up, the animal was marked with a "T" on its jaw and sent to slaughter. TB was a big concern, because it could be easily spread. The distance to the slaughterhouse was some 30 miles, near where the Albany airport is now, and the animals had to travel by foot. Many were not able to make it. Some of the cows were old—kept in the herd as "Ma" cows to nurse calves on—or had poor feet. We had an old lineback cow, about 16 years old, which reacted positive to the test. She was a nice cow, with a white line down her back, and my mother had raised her from a calf. She was kind of special—small, but she gave a lot of milk.

When my mother learned that the cow would have to walk all that way to slaughter, it was the first time that I saw her and the other farm ladies band together in protest. They telephoned one another and rallied for a better way to get the cattle transported. The women agreed that the cattle needed to go, but they shouldn't have to walk the entire distance. I remember there was quite a fury over it. My mother said, "If the older cows have to go, then take them by truck." The state responded to the protest and hired a truck to transport the animals that couldn't make the journey on foot.

I rode along on horseback and helped to lead the cattle well enough to walk on the route to Albany. I would have been 10 years old then, and remember that early April morning when the ground was still snowy. My job was to keep the cows off of everyone's lawn and alert the people ahead. Most properties had a fence around them at that time, which made my job easier.

The men drove the cattle down Goode Street and Lakehill Road to the flagpole, and took a right to go down through the south part of Burnt Hills. It started out as a small group, but we added more cows from farms along the way. We went over the railroad tracks and across the bridge over the Mohawk River to the Rickmyer's farm on the other side. That's as far as we went. At this point, someone else took over leading the group forward, covering the total distance to the slaughterhouse in three days.

TB tests were done every few years, and the next test after the pill was a tuberculine liquid in a syringe, which was injected near the cow's tail. Some bulls reacted positive and went to slaughter too. Everyone got paid for their losses— state and federal inspectors came, along with a meat appraiser, and purebred cattle brought more money than grades. One farmer near us, who had a small herd of Guernseys, lost seven cows the first time TB tests were administered. The second time his herd was tested, he had so few cows left that he told the inspectors to just take them all because he was going out of business.

EARNING MONEY

When I was about 12 I had my first business venture raising chickens. It was during the Depression, and there wasn't much money. Things were pretty tight, but my dad signed for me to borrow $500 from the Ballston Bank, and we bought 500 day-old baby chicks. These were Rhode Island Reds in straight runs, meaning that there were males as well as females. When the roosters got big enough, we would sell them for meat, and that would give me a payment for the bank. By the time the pullets were ready to lay, we'd have some more to sell. We had one big brooder house, and put two coal burners in there. I had a cot in the middle and I slept with them—that's how much I was worried about paying that money back to the bank! We didn't lose many of the chicks and continued to raise a new crop of baby chickens each year for three years. We did a lot of business with the Barber and Bennett Feed Company in Albany. Their feed salesman, Charlie, would come and advise me on what to give the chickens, and they bought shelled ear corn from us.

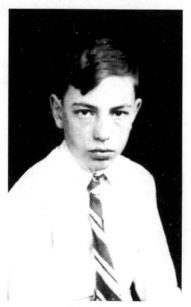

Serious Business!

While I was in the chicken business, Dick Brown, a local carpenter and painter, told me about a home remedy to get rid of the lice on my birds. I went down to Dave Bayliss' barbershop where they had a cuspidor. Everything went into that besides the tobacco juice—even cigar butts. I asked Mr. Bayliss what he did with that mess when he emptied it, and he said, "I put it on my roses." I asked him if he would save me some in a bottle to put on my chicken roost. One afternoon Dick and I cleaned off the roost, painted the nicotine sulfate on with a feather, and lined the floor with newspapers underneath. When the chickens flew up on the roost, within minutes the lice were down on the bottom. We just pulled the paper out quickly and burned it. You could buy stuff called "Black Leaf Forty," which was the same thing except much more expensive, but our homemade nicotine sulfate worked just fine.

Another moneymaking venture for me was catching woodchucks. Woodchucks were a problem on the farm—they'd get in the fencerow and then make holes in the fields. If a horse stepped into a hole while cutting hay it could break a leg. My dad said, "If you want to catch those woodchucks, I'll give you 25¢ for every one you get." I started out trapping, and I might have gotten two or three a day, but then I got kind of inventive. I went down to the gas station in Burnt Hills and found an old rubber hose that was frazzled on the end. The floorboards on the Model T lifted up, so I put the hose on the exhaust, and ran the other end into the woodchuck hole. I started with gas and then switched to kerosene—it smoked great. I was getting five or six woodchucks out of each hole! I was really making money then! Well, I pulled the choke too many times, and the Model-T caught on fire. I got scared and decided to run it through the pond by the barns.

When I got home, I was ready for the lickin' of my life. My dad had a razor strap that hung up higher than I could reach. The girls used to get a swat with it, and Melvin did too, but I hardly ever got it being the youngest. My folks would just look at it, and I could see what was coming. But when it came to bringing the truck home on fire, my mother said, "You know this time you're going to get it." Before my dad got home, I put on (underneath a pair of coveralls) the leather guards that Melvin wore when he rode his motorcycle. My dad felt bad when he used the strap on me that day—I wasn't enjoying it, but I wasn't hurting either.

THE GOODE "STREET"

Although my family had lived at our farm since 1911, our road was still in pretty bad shape in the 1930's. One night in February, J.B. White got his car stuck in the ruts and snow so he walked up our lane and rapped on the door. This happened at around 9:30 at night and my dad had gone to bed. My mother was still up canning some meat, and J.B. asked her, "Would Dave be around? My car is stuck on the road and I wonder if he would pull me out." My father got out of bed, harnessed up the horses, and dragged the chain and clevis down our lane through the snow. After my dad got him out, J.B. asked, "Well, Dave, what do I owe you?" My father replied, "How about three dollars?" J.B. said that he only had a hundred dollar bill on him. My dad said, "That's all right," and dug into his pocket to count out ninety-seven dollars in change.

That's how he operated back then, my dad always kept the money he had in his pocket. When my mother needed to get groceries, she got a $20 bill from him. I remember the bills used to be yellow then. If we were justified in spending some money, and could explain where it was needed, he would hand some out.

My Uncle Bert Garrison was the Supervisor in the Town of Ballston. In the early fall of an election year he would hold a caucus down in Burnt Hills—usually at Turpit's store on the south street. Uncle Bert asked my dad, "Dave, what can we do for the farmers down there in your area?" My dad told him, "I wish you could get the road fixed. It's been bad since we moved here." Besides the terrible ruts, the road was low, and the bushes and stone walls on the west side of the road created snow drifts in the winter. Uncle Bert came through and the road crew cut the brush, put the stones through a crusher, and raised the road. It was quite an improvement, and that's how it became Goode Street instead of Goode Road. For years after that, a woman named Ellen Winters, who was the Town Highway Superintendent would say to me, "Keep the road up and the ditches low."

ADVANCES IN FARMING

The first county agent I remember was Hank Little, who came out of Cornell, and started the Extension Service in Saratoga County. Hank was a tall, lanky fellow who always wore a full-brimmed hat. He loved to come and talk with the farmers, and was interested in helping any young person

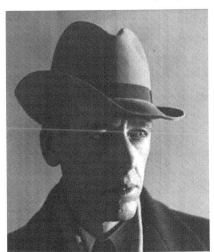

Harold B. Little
Photo Courtesy of Cornell Cooperative Extension
Records Management / Archives

who might follow in his footsteps and go to Cornell. The older people weren't sure about his new ideas for farming and sort of backed off. Hank didn't get through to my dad very quickly either. He advised my dad and Mr. Merchant, who had the farm just north of us, to introduce more alfalfa instead of growing just timothy and other kinds of grass hay. He also encouraged them to test their ground to see what the pH level of the soil was. They found out it ought to be around seven in order to grow alfalfa. Hank told them if they applied lime at two tons to the acre, they'd get four times as much hay, and three cuttings off the fields. That was never talked about before Hank came, so my dad, Steve Merchant and a few other farmers decided to buy a carload of lime. When the train came into Ballston Lake the car had to be unloaded within 72 hours. The only way to get the loads home was with the sleigh, so the town highway crew left snow for us on one half of Lakehill Road, and just plowed the other half. After seeing how the lime worked, and getting twice the cuttings and yield of hay, some farmers in the area were a lot more open to new ways of doing things.

One spring, a stranger came walking up our lane, and saw our mares and foals in the pasture. He leaned on the fence just watching them until my dad came out from the house. It was about the time when we really needed some help—Melvin was getting married and starting the apprentice course at G.E. so he wouldn't be around much anymore. This man, whose name was Bob Goldie, had come from Schenectady on the Welcome Bus Line (this bus was also called the Irish Kate) and got off in Burnt Hills. We thought that he was probably headed up to Knight's or Merchant's to look for work, and just stopping to admire the horses. It turns out he didn't know squat about farming, but asked my Dad for a job anyhow. You can imagine how hard it was to find help. We did not know Bob Goldie and he didn't know us, but he became a great friend. He adopted all the horses and the cows, and stayed with us for 10 years.

Bob Goldie was inclined to be quite a drinker and a smoker, so my father sat him down and had a talk. He told him if he wanted to work at our farm, he couldn't be smoking in the barn. We had an old milkcan out there for his cigarette butts, and he kept his smoking outside. He took time off about once a month to visit his sister in Schenectady and soak up some of the city. That held him over for a while, but when the Watkins Man came around with veterinary supplies, he'd drink that damn liniment! He really was good help, and was always there when we needed him for threshing, cutting ice, and any of the other jobs on the farm. The day my dad died, Bob Goldie told my mother he couldn't work for anybody else, and then he left.

DAD DIES

I was 16 when my dad died in February of 1935; it felt like the world had suddenly come right down on top of me. He was never sick a day in his life, but had been having some trouble urinating. His doctor scheduled prostate surgery, and as it turned out, Dad was admitted into the hospital when my mother was away on a nursing call. He thought he'd be out in a day or two when my mother would be back home. Other than the prostate problem he was perfectly healthy and strong as he could be when he went in. I visited Dad in the hospital after the surgery, but soon after, the family was informed that a blood clot had caused him to have a stroke. They didn't follow today's practices of thinning the blood or getting the patient up and moving back then. He was 71 years old.

My dad's death was a traumatic blow and devastating loss but there was nothing else we could do but pick ourselves up and carry on. Somehow my mother and I managed to pull things together to run the farm, and I finished my sophomore year of high school that spring. There were a lot of people that came to help, and who became positive influences in the decisions I made from that point on.

Melvin, who was living in Schenectady with his wife, came home to help out on the farm whenever he had time, and Steve Merchant, Sr., who I often referred to as Father Merchant, came down several times and rode on the 1020 tractor. "I've been going by here watching you plow," he'd say, "You're doing a great job." Stephen Merchant was the first farmer in Saratoga County to earn the honor of "Master Farmer" in New York State, and advised me on a lot of things.

At that time, we had so much old machinery that we were lucky to get a crop in. We had an old grain drill with wooden wheels and metal rims. In order to use it we had to back it into the pond to let the wheels swell. We thought, "there's got to be a better way to farm it than this," and realized how much we needed to upgrade.

Dr. Harry Hansen, the veterinarian, came down after Dad died. He had gotten to know my father pretty well, and had a lot of respect for him, so I called Harry whenever I had a sick animal. Harry was one of the few people I had talked to about becoming a veterinarian, and I guess I believed it could be possible, but I had no idea it would ever come true. I couldn't imagine how to even begin to follow this dream with no money, and the reality of managing the farm bearing down on me. I stayed with our cows that were going to have a calf, and with some of our mares that were going to have a foal. My mother was in the house, but there was nobody else around. I learned a lot about birthing. Sometimes the animals needed my help, but I didn't touch them if I didn't have to.

Frank Stevens, my science teacher (who later became the Principal), and Ray Benjamin, my basketball and cross-country coach, were also great mentors after my dad passed away. They brought some senior students with them to the farm that summer and helped us with the hay. I can remember Frank coming in a pair of shorts—by the end of the day there were so many red spots and scratches on his legs from handling the bales of hay, he looked like he had the chicken pox!

Frank Stevens thought there were two of us in the class of 1937 who would possibly go on to college. I hadn't planned on ever going when my dad was alive, but I soon realized that things had changed. Farm work was becoming mechanical, and everything on our farm needed to be updated. There was just too much to do, so I thought more about college and becoming a veterinarian than I ever had before.

I never could have continued my education without Frank Stevens' encouragement. None of my siblings had gotten through high school, and it was quite a challenge for me to think that I could do it. My mother said if I could find extra help to do the farm work she was all for it.

Hank Little, the county agent who had gone to Cornell, was also an inspiration in getting me to go on to school. He was the kind of man who was looking to help young people get ahead.

In addition to thinking about my own future, I was also concerned about my mother. Her health started to decline after my dad died and she worried about what would become of the farm. She wanted to stay there for the rest of her days, but some members of my family were more inclined to sell the farm. I started to think that if I didn't hurry up and buy it, there'd be no farm left. We let things stay as they were for a few years, and I continued with high school and work-ing the farm.

In 11th grade I was elected president of the class, not because I knew that much, but I guess my teachers wanted to make sure I finished high school—if I was involved, I would be more likely to stick with it. Around that time, my mother said she wouldn't make any more pants with cuffs for me, because they were always full of sawdust, silage and hay. Sometimes I forgot to dump the cuffs out, and they'd get soggy and the pants would be ruined. At school we were

48

called the "hicks"—the Knight's, Merchant's, Jenkins' and me—because we didn't have cuffs on our pants, but we didn't mind. The boys at Ballston Lake were called the "branch boys" because they lived near the junction of the train tracks and worked unloading the cars. There was a lot of friction between the Burnt Hills boys and the Ballston Lake boys. We all started playing basketball together though and eventually got to know each other, becoming good friends.

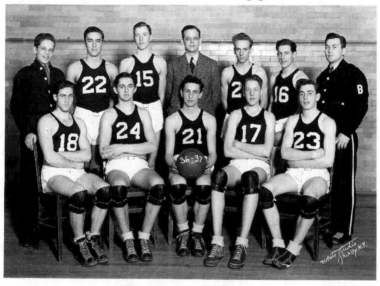

BH-BL BASKETBALL TEAM 1936-37
Front Row (L-R) Sam Benjamin, Jim Yates, Lou Eger,
Norman Lamb, Stan Garrison. Back Row (L-R) Fred Foss,
Melvin Smith, Don Wait, Principal Fred Crum, Donald Flicker,
Walt Morris, and Coach Ray Benjamin.

Frank Stevens thought Andy Caldwell and I would be the two from our class to go to college. We were probably just marginal students, but Andy was better than I was. Frank said, "I think we'll have to give you boys a short course in chemistry, so you'll be able to meet the requirements for college when you go." Frank and his wife, Mabel, had just gotten married and lived down in Ballston Lake. Frank set up a Saturday morning for us to come down to his house, and he put on a demonstration to explain how a catalyst worked. Mabel went next door to the little camps on the east side of the lake, so we had the house to ourselves. Frank was going to make biscuits and show us how they would rise when baking powder was added. Well it went the other way—the biscuits dropped and had a hole in the middle. The house was filled with smoke, and Frank stuffed the biscuits full of strawberry jam for us to eat. We still got into college anyway.

We had my group of Boy Scouts at the farm one night—this was after my father had passed away. Someone thought that the smokehouse would be a good place to take the fire-starting course, so two of the boys went in and started a fire. Unbeknownst to them, there was dynamite stored in the top of the building. My mother was probably the one who caught on and immediately alerted the Scouts of the danger. The dynamite didn't go off, but the thought of what could have happened that night sure scared us for a while.

I can remember going to get my first hunting license at about that time. There was no town office then, and Gene Murray was the Town Clerk of Charlton. When I was leaving his place he told me to help myself to some of his muskmelons just outside the door. He had a nice patch of melons, so I took one home. The next night was a Saturday. Earl Wetsel, Albert Merchant and I went by the melon patch, and picked up a few of those melons to eat—they were so good. We took one apiece, and brought the melons up to a dance in Charlton, where Gene Murray was taking the tickets. We told Gene we didn't have any money, but we had three muskmelons, so he said, "Just put 'em in the basket and we'll sell 'em here," and he gave us three tickets in exchange.

MEETING SHIRLEY

Over the years I've learned that fate has an awful lot to do with some things. Mrs. Brown, my math teacher, had a message for me and she asked Shirley Miller to deliver it. Shirley was in 9th grade and I was a senior. Our school was spread out with the gym and cafeteria on the ground level, and two floors upstairs. The senior class was meeting in the farthest room back on the second floor. Because I was class President, I was standing up in front of the room, while we were talking about earning money for our class trip. Shirley was terrified, but came way down the big hall, tapped on the door, and handed me the piece of paper. This was the first time she had an inkling of who I was, and the first time I caught sight of her. So I read the note from "Ma" Brown, which said she would help me upgrade my marks in math, but I didn't care about math right then. I was more interested in seeing Shirley. As I stepped out of the room the whole class let out a squeal. I can remember Shirley going back down that long hall with her plaid skirt swaying. She got to the other end and looked back. I didn't know whether a senior could date a freshman or not, and thought I had better wait for her to grow up a little bit.

My friend Dick White's girlfriend, Eleanor, was in my class, and wanted to go to the prom. Dick didn't know how to dance, so he asked me if I would take her. I told him that I would show him how to dance instead. Well, he didn't learn the steps very well and wasn't comfortable going to the prom. Eleanor was a nice gal, and Dick talked me into taking her after all. She lived at the top of the hill on Hetcheltown Road, where her father grew hundreds of tomato plants. On the night of the prom, the temperature dropped, so we had to leave the prom and help her dad put hot caps on all those tomato plants. We both had boots on, and Eleanor was still in her long gown—we were quite a sight.

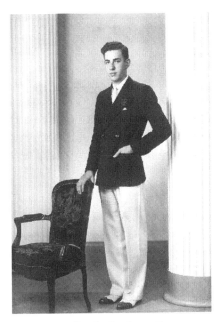

All "decked out"

Before we graduated, our senior class made it to Washington, D.C., for our class trip. There were 30 of us that went. It was tight, but we earned enough money to go by doing odd jobs, and cleaning up around Burnt Hills. We all worked hard to make our town look good, and the whole community chipped in. The Washington trip was a yearly event, and our senior class was excited to take in all the sights of the monuments and even a play while we were there. It was the biggest city most of us had ever seen.

Graduation exercises for the class of 1937 were held on the lawn in front of the school, and Thomas Denny, president of the school board, handed out the diplomas. This was a big day for me, and I know my mother was especially proud. I wish that my dad could have been there to share it with her and and the rest of our family.

After high school my mother and I continued to run the farm together. The following year we bought a new Ford

Ferguson, which was the first tractor we owned with rubber tires. It was quite a thing back then. Before that, we had a 1020 that could shake your kidneys loose when you drove it.

I had priced the tractor, and was about to buy it from Dick White, who worked for Carl King's dealership. For taking his girlfriend Eleanor to the prom, and helping him sell three more tractors, Dick agreed to take some money off the price of the Ford Ferguson. I got the tractor and 14" hydraulic plows for $825.

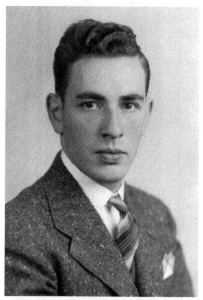

Stan, an enterprising young man

That little tractor fit the bill on our farm, and I used it for many projects in our area too. One time I planted 40 acres of buckwheat at the Schenectady County Airport in Glenville, and my nephew, Alton, combined it for me. In the winter I used the snowplow and tractor to plow out a lot of businesses in Burnt Hills and down Route 50 to Sarnowski's dairy, then in to Broadway in Schenectady to do Max Cohen's market. It could get pretty chilly on this little tractor without a cab!

Seeing all the planes come and go while planting buckwheat at the airport sparked my interest in flying, and I decided to take lessons there. The flight instructor would regularly ask me if I had cleaned my shoes before we got in the plane together. He was worried that with the heat of the engines the smell of cow manure would fill that little cockpit. I did my ground-school work at Union College, and passed my flight test by making a last minute decision in the air. The weather had been clear when we left the airport in Scotia the day of my test, but when we reached Glens Falls, there was six inches of new snow on the ground. I circled the field twice and decided to fly to Troy where I landed the plane and filed a new flight plan. It was the safe thing to do, and the instructor said I had passed.

Around the time I took up flying, my sister Anna Mae, and her husband Phil Pashley, bought the old District 8 schoolhouse on Route 50. Everyone called it "Dizzy 8". The state was planning to straighten the road, and the schoolhouse needed to be moved, so I helped my sister's husband do this. I cut some hickory logs to put under the building for skids, and at five o'clock in the morning, using my little tractor and loader, we brought that little schoolhouse across Route 50 and down Pashley Road about 500 yards. We didn't have a permit or anything, and figured it was easier if we just got the job done.

I came back to Pashley Road that spring to plow my sister's garden, and ended up meeting Mrs. Miller, my future mother-in-law. The Millers lived across the road from my sister, and I backed into their ditch to unload my tractor and plow. When Mrs. Miller saw me, she asked if I would plow her garden too, so I did. That was a few years before I began dating Shirley—the woman I would marry.

In 1938, when I was 20 years old, I went to see Morgan Welch, President of the Ballston Bank. I wanted to get a loan to buy the farm. It was a tough time to buy a farm, but a good time to buy one. With the economy as it was then the price would never be any lower, but without enough equity in the farm the bank would be skeptical about taking the risk. Laura and Melvin wanted me to own it, so we had the farm appraised to know what it was worth. Mr. Welch said he'd like to make the loan, but bank policy required that borrowers be at least 21 years of age. He knew that I had faithfully paid off the loans each spring for my chickens when I was a boy, but that was back when my dad was alive, and signed the papers for me. Officially, I didn't have any credit of my own. Mr. Welch thought for a minute and said there might be a way to borrow the money after all. If I could find somebody to sign the note, the bank might take a chance on me.

I suggested to Mr. Welch, "How about Bert Garrison?" He thought that was a fine idea, and advised that we call him. Bert was my uncle, and had been the Town Supervisor. He agreed to sign for me so I could borrow the money. That was a turning point in my life. To be able to buy our farm with just a signature from Uncle Bert was like a dream come true. Uncle Bert knew it was a valuable farm, but probably never would have signed the papers if he'd known I was about to go to college. Then again, I didn't know I was going to go either, but that's how it turned out.

CORNELL WINTER COURSE

Sometimes you happen to be in the right place at the right time. I remember the county agent, Hank Little, encouraging me to go to Cornell. He said, "If you can't go for the whole year, then just go for the Winter Course." I told my mother, "I'd like to go and find out what classes I'd need to become a veterinarian." She answered, "If you can find someone to stay here at the farm and do the chores, that would be fine." The Winter Course at Cornell went from November through February. Vince Plummer, a young man who helped with haying during the summer, came and stayed with my mother during those months, and said he had the time of his life because she fed him so good! My nephew Alton helped Vince that winter too.

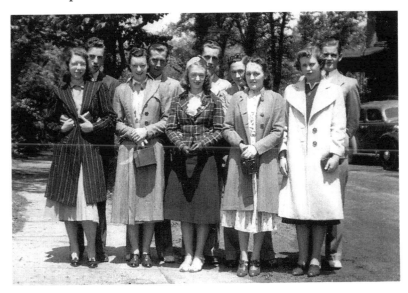

Local friends visiting us in Ithaca
Winter Course at Cornell University 1938-39
(L-R) Bernice Bubb, Stan Garrison, Etta Larkin, Albert Merchant,
Rosemary Casey, Earl Wetsel, Russell Robinson,
Minnie Boswell, Myrna VanPatten and Vernon Fobian.

I went out to Cornell with Frank Holbrook, Woody Arnold, and Emmor Caldwell, who were all local farmers like myself. We lived together in Ithaca, took some good agricultural courses, and I also learned what was required to enter the New York State College of Veterinary Medicine at Cornell.

One weekend that winter, Frank and I brought Woody home to attend his brother's wedding. When we left to head back to Ithaca on Sunday the snow was blowing and drifting so bad that we got stuck on Route 20 in the town of Pompey. We decided to wait out the storm, and as there was no hotel nearby, we were thankful that a kind resident in town took us in to stay overnight. I was recovering from a hernia operation at the time, so Woody and Frank shared the double bed while I slept on the sofa. It was so cold during the night that all three of us crowded together in the bed to stay warm. The next morning we found out that another student, who was also stranded, had slept in the bathtub. The plows came through to clear the roads, and we were all back on our way.

While I was attending the Winter Course, Dr. Winfield Stone, a 1935 graduate of the Veterinary College at Cornell, befriended me. He advised me to get one year of college as a pre-vet student before applying to Cornell because they were changing the curriculum and I would need the background.

DATING SHIRLEY

That spring of 1939, I took Shirley to her junior prom, and we dated throughout her senior year of high school. Evidently I remembered her more than she remembered me. I could still picture that shy girl in the plaid skirt who had handed me a note two years earlier. Money was tight so we did things that didn't cost a lot like ice skating, or going to the community dances at the hall in Ballston Lake. Occasionally, we went bowling or rollerskating in Schenectady or to a movie in Ballston. I think that my sister, Anna Mae, and her neighbor, Mrs. Miller, had a lot to do with bringing Shirley and me back together.

During Shirley's senior year of high school, I took a year of college courses to get ready for vet school. My mother was in poor health, but she wanted to see me continue on with my education if I could. I went to Siena, a Catholic College. Father Hogan, a well-known priest from Our Lady of Grace Church in Ballston Lake, got me in. At that time there were no Protestant boys at Siena. The college had just started a few years before, but I was admitted as the 40th student in the pre-med group in 1939. Father Ben was my math teacher, and also a man who loved to eat. I took him to some of the church suppers in our community, and he would tell the greatest stories.

On Thursdays at Siena, I had a light day of classes, which allowed me to deliver eggs from our farm to Albany. It was then that I got to know Dr. Ivan Howe, head of the Department of Agriculture and Markets for New York State. Dr. Howe took an interest in me because I had the farm, and his 12-year-old son wanted to become a veterinarian too. He kept me posted on what was going on at Cornell, and when a new class might be starting at the Veterinary College.

Dr. Howe was a wonderful person to know and, years later, informed me of a purebred Hereford sale at the Karker Ranch in Warnerville, N.Y. I went to look at the cows and brought my nephew Alton with me. Alton had always wanted to visit a ranch out West, and stayed to work at the Karker Ranch for the summer. Prior to the sale, I wound up buying eight Hereford cows ready to freshen, and brought them home.

When the day of the sale came around for the rest of the herd, I met the owners of the Karker Ranch. Mr. Herbert Taylor was one of the partners, and he had learned of my interest in becoming a veterinarian. He asked if I knew Dr.

58

William Hagan, Dean at the Cornell Veterinary College. Mr. Taylor and Dean Hagan had been best friends while in college at Northwestern University in Evanston, Illinois, in the early 1900's. Mr. Taylor also asked if I was familiar with an organization called Rotary. I did not know Dean Hagan; nor did I know about Rotary. Our meeting was fateful. Mr. Herbert Taylor would later influence my life more than I could have imagined at that time. He wrote a note to his friend, Dean Hagan on my behalf. Mr. Taylor also went on to develop the famous four-way test, the code of ethics adopted by Rotary clubs worldwide. In 1953 he became President of Rotary International.

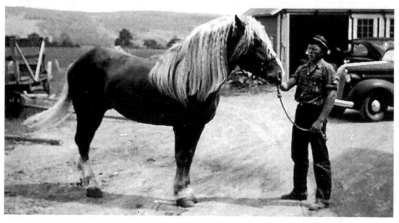

My nephew, Alton Close, with a Belgian draft horse at the Karker Ranch, Warnerville, N.Y.

Another coincidence the day of that cattle sale at Karker Ranch involved Dr. Walter Kessler. He gave the invocation before the barbecue and, years later, I got to know him when he became the minister of the Methodist Church in Burnt Hills.

I made many valuable contacts while at Siena College, and finished up the year with good marks—much better than my grades from high school. Siena was good to me.

SHIRLEY GRADUATES AND MY MOTHER DIES

I didn't make it to Shirley's high school graduation in June of 1940. I was the only one home when my mother passed away that same night. I would have liked to have heard Shirley's speech; she was valedictorian of her class despite having attended seven different schools! That was quite an accomplishment. Shirley's father was a carpenter during the Depression and her family moved many times, to wherever he could find work. The Miller family finally settled in East Glenville when Shirley started 8th grade. She liked journalism and became editor of the school paper.

When my mother died, some of the friars from Siena came to her funeral in their big black car. They didn't have to come, but they did, and it made me feel good to realize how much other people cared when I had just lost someone so close to me.

Shirley came up to the house after the funeral and saw the kitchen sink…that dishpan was just full! I can't tell you how many cans of Spam I ate back then. Shirley washed up the dishes, and I was especially grateful.

G.E.

With my mother gone and my year at Siena finished, I decided to take a job at General Electric, and continue farming on the side. After graduation, Shirley had gotten a job at the G.E. as well. I sold the milk cows and raised beef cattle and crops, while working the second shift as a machinist. The boss was a friend of my sister Laura's, and I was glad he put me to work on the line rather than having me take the machinist's course. I told him that I intended to apply to Cornell when the war was over, and he understood that my position was only temporary.

It was then that I got my draft notice. I knew some people in Albany and told them I had my pilot's license to fly small planes, but they needed pilots who could fly the bigger planes to transport soldiers. They suggested that I continue working the farm and at my job at G.E.

Meat was scarce during the war, and the big boss at G.E. asked if I would sell one of my Hereford beef cows. He came to the farm and picked out the one that he wanted, which probably weighed 1400 pounds on the hoof. Beef cows usually dress out at half their live weight, but this one weighed about 200 pounds per quarter! Shirley helped me with the butchering, and I let it hang overnight in quarters. The next morning, I backed up the truck, and took the beef to a friend's cooler in Schenectady to be processed.

WEDDING BELLS

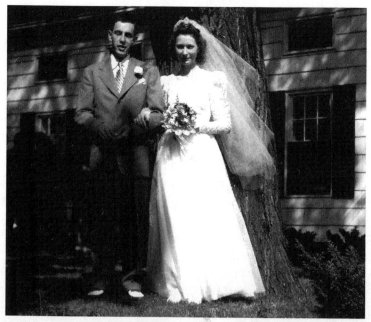

Our Wedding Reception at the Millers' Home

On Shirley's birthday in May of 1941, we had dinner at her parent's house and I gave her an engagement ring. Afterwards we went to Dutcher's with my sister Laura and her boyfriend for an ice cream sundae to celebrate our engagement.

We were engaged for a year, and got married May 30th, 1942. Shirley wanted a center aisle for the wedding, so we had it at the Baptist Church in Burnt Hills. We had two ministers to perform the ceremony: a Baptist from that church, Rev. Briggs, and a Methodist, Rev. White, from the church that my family usually attended. Lou Eger, my friend and former captain of our basketball team, was best man, and Dot Miller, Shirley's sister-in-law, was matron of honor. Shirley's niece was the flower girl, and my nephew was ring bearer.

On the farm it seemed that there was never enough time to get everything done. Shirley said that I was even late for our wedding! In the days leading up to our big day, I was busy planting corn. There was rationing due to the war, but we had enough gas in our blue Ford to get us started on our three day honeymoon. We drove north as far as Port Henry, where a friend's son got us coupons for a couple of cans of gas. We went to dinner in Elizabethtown, stayed at a little hotel in Lewis, and drove into Canada the next day. In Montreal we found a nice hotel, and in the morning we walked up the street to a restaurant for breakfast. Everybody in town stared Shirley down because she was wearing slacks. I guess it wasn't yet acceptable for women to wear pants there in 1942! On our way back home, we stayed a night in Lake Placid, but then had to get home to finish planting corn.

When Shirley and I were first married, I was still working the second shift at G.E. This meant that Shirley was alone during the afternoons and all evening until midnight. There was nobody else around for company at our farmhouse and big old barn except for the dog. I kept one cow that was an easy milker, and Shirley had to go down to the barn and milk the cow at night. One time when we found a horse harness all cut up in the woods, Shirley was scared to death—she thought some crazy person was running around with a butcher knife!

We had three brooder houses full of small chickens that year, and about 100 of them got smothered when wind from a storm blew the big door in and it fell on them. We were short of money, and rather than bury them, we cut the heads off and Shirley hung the chickens on the clothesline! Early the next morning, we loaded them in the truck and took them to the chicken shack on Broadway, where we got a dollar apiece for them, feathers and all.

That summer of '42 was the last year we had the threshers come to separate the grain from the straw and chaff. We changed works with the neighbors, and when it was our turn, ten farmers came to thresh the oats at our farm. Shirley had never cooked for a crowd, and her father was remodeling our kitchen at the time. We had ordered an electric stove, but had to wait a month to get it because of the war, so all that Shirley had to cook on was a hot plate! Luckily, Shirley's mother was a good cook, and helped her to feed all those hungry men. Shirley said her mother really saved the day, and that she didn't know what she would have done without her.

I continued working my job at G.E. to supplement our income from the farm. It was a good job at that time and the company even gave us a war bond when our first daughter, Diane, was born in November of 1943. Shirley took care of our little family, and helped me send inquiry letters to 18 veterinary colleges including one in Guelph, Ontario! The responses were all the same—there would be no new classes until the war was over.

In the early 1940's, our veterinarian, Dr. Harry Hansen, wrote a letter to his good friend, Dr. Myron Fincher, at

Cornell University. Harry had graduated from the Veterinary College at Cornell in 1932. He told Dr. Fincher that he knew a young fellow who had finished pre-med classes at Siena College, and would like to become a veterinarian. Dr. Fincher was soon named Acting Dean of the College of Veterinary Medicine, replacing his superior, Dr. Hagan, who was needed for the Marshall Plan. There had been a terrible outbreak of Hoof and Mouth disease in Europe and research at Plum Island (located off the northeastern tip of Long Island) was being conducted to prevent its spread to the U.S.

It wasn't until the summer of 1945 when I was up on a 50-foot ladder, painting near the peak of the roof on the big barn that I heard anything about veterinary school. Shirley came out to where I was working and shouted up, "There's a car here with a Cornell insignia on it!" So down I came off the ladder—and don't you think it wasn't pretty quick. Dr. Fincher and Dr. Baker, who were both veterinary professors at Cornell, were on their way to the yearling sales in Saratoga. They had stopped to see Dr. Harry Hansen in Ballston, and then drove down to our place. Shirley brought us some tea and cookies and our visitors felt right at home. She really made an impression. Before they left, Dr. Fincher said to me, "Come on out to Cornell, and I'll give you an interview next Tuesday at 10 a.m." You can imagine at that moment I felt as if God had just touched me on the shoulder. I had waited a long time for something like that to happen!

The following Tuesday we left Diane with Shirley's mother, and went to Ithaca for the interview. Dr. Fincher talked to both Shirley and me, saying that going to school and being married wasn't going to be easy for either of us. This didn't bother us though. We received a letter in the mail two weeks later saying that finally I had been accepted. There had been 1100 applicants to the program, and only 46 chosen for our class—40 veterans, five non-veterans, and one woman. As I look back, I know the chances of my getting in weren't the greatest. I think that more than anything, I was accepted because of Harry's letter to Dr. Fincher and the personal visit that summer. I've always believed that fate had a lot to do with it. If I hadn't been painting the barn that day and missed Dr. Fincher, I don't know what would have happened. I know Shirley impressed them more than my marks!

This was all great news, but there was a lot to do! In just a few months time I would have to give up my job at G.E., sell the Herefords, rent our farmhouse, figure out where we'd live in Ithaca, and how we'd pay our bills!

ITHACA, NEW YORK–1945

Because the war had just ended, and there were so many returning veterans, our class at veterinary college didn't start until October of 1945. I was 27 then, and we were all older than the typical first-year students; 30 of us out of 46 were married and had children. I have to give credit to the wives of my classmates (as well as my own!) Anyone looking at that class would know it was a strain on our young families. Nobody had any money, but we got together with other couples and played cards, or went on picnics; we made some wonderful friends that we still keep in touch with. My classmates came from all over the country, not very many from New York State.

The one woman in our class, whose name was Jean Holzworth, was an exceptional student. She was my lab partner, since Holzworth followed Garrison alphabetically. She helped me with the bookwork, and I helped her with the practical part. I wasn't the smartest one in our class, and had to repeat a few courses, but I got through. Jean went on to write many books, and has probably done more research on feline diseases than anyone.

Another classmate and friend, Lyle Baker, had been in a prison camp during the war. He showed us the diary he had kept, which was shocking to read. He was married, and he and his wife Barbara were very close friends of ours. Lyle was 10 years ahead of everybody with his research on cows' nutrition, believing many diseases could be corrected by feeding cattle the proper diet.

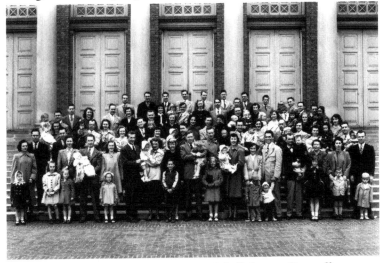

NYS College of Veterinary Medicine at Cornell
Class of 1950 with their spouses and children

In our very first class we were told, "You are starting out with 46 in your class, but six weeks from now, there will only be 40 of you here." It was probably true, but I was determined to be among the 40 who stayed, especially after all that it had taken to get there! Dr. Francis Fox, who taught a lot of the practical classes, including physical diagnosis, was one of the people I looked up to. Dr. Fox was five years younger than me—imagine him teaching our class of older students! His supervisor was Dr. Myron Fincher, one of the professors who visited us that summer. They both had offices upstairs, above the classrooms in the medical building. People who knew him well called Dr. Fincher "Mike". In that medical building they also had a black cat named Mike. Every once in a while, when Dr.

Fox was teaching downstairs, the cat would make a noise overhead. He'd holler up, "Mike, come on down here!" and Dr. Fincher would look over the rail and ask, "Are you talking to me, Dr. Fox?"

I discovered early on in my studies that I liked genetics—it was a subject I was pretty good in. One day in class, Dr. F.B. Hutt, our genetics professor, showed us a hundred pictures of different breeds of animals on the screen, and we had to identify them. He bet that no one would know over 70 of them. If someone did, he said that person wouldn't have to take the class. I scored over 70 on the test, but wanted to take the course anyway.

Dr. Donald Baker was the man who came to the farm with Dr. Fincher that summer on their way to Saratoga. We called him "Bugs" Baker because he was always monkeying with the insects. He got us some microscopes from WWII that had three oculars, and a wooden case for just three dollars. I used that little microscope for years.

While I got along well with most of my professors, I had a rough start with Dr. Pete Olafson. He had a look that could burn a hole right through you, and he didn't smile very much. On the occasions that he did smile, I got an inkling that maybe I'd given him the right answer to a question he didn't expect me to get. Early on, I remember him saying to me "How the hell did you get in here?" Dr. Olafson wasn't involved in the selection process for student admissions and I suspected that he might have had some other candidates in mind for the limited availability of slots. He was the head of Pathology and I thought, "If he doesn't think I'm very smart, I'll offer to help him"—so I did the setup for the next class each day, and worked for him in Post Mortem. He got to like me pretty well, and when I was ready to graduate in 1950 he said, "What are you going to do with yourself now? I suppose you'd like to be President of the State Veterinary Society." I said, "Yes, I'd like to do that. Just give me 20 years." (And it was 1971 when I began my term.)

There was housing on campus for the veterans—clusters of small homes built on Tower Road called "Vetsburg." If you were not a veteran but had children like me, it was difficult to find an apartment. So Shirley and I bought an old house trailer in Vermont, packed it with canned goods and started off with it to Ithaca before school started. The first tire blew on a big hill past Fort Plain, and when we got to Cortland we got another flat. Tires were scarce, and so were trailer parks at that time. We ended up parking it in somebody's yard in the town of Varna. There we were with a two-year old, and me trying to study, after years of being away from the books. We had no running water and used an outhouse on the property. We soon decided that the trailer wasn't going to work. Shirley was expecting our second child then, so she and Diane went back home to Burnt Hills, and I stayed at the Alpha Psi fraternity house on Elmwood Avenue.

In June of 1946, when I returned home, our daughter Linda was born. We cropped the fields every summer to earn money for my next year of college, and sold the oats, wheat or rye to the Barber and Bennett Company in Albany. When I bought our farm in Burnt Hills, it didn't seem like the thing to do at the time, but Shirley and I look back now and know that's how we got through my time at Cornell.

The following fall we bought a 55-acre farm in Danby, just outside of Ithaca. It wasn't much, but provided us with a place to live. We built an apartment on the second story of our farmhouse, took in some boarders, and I went to work part-time at the Large Animal Clinic while going to school. We even cropped some of the land at the new farm with a pair of Belgian fillies. Eventually we sold this team of horses to a retired man in Etna who wanted to deliver groceries. We ate a lot of eggs in Danby since the lady at the farm next door sold us the cracked ones for next to nothing. We lived there for three years before selling the place to the man who had been renting the apartment.

In 1948, while we were in Ithaca, Shirley's parents sold their house on Pashley Road, and moved to our farm on Goode Street in Burnt Hills. No one was living in our farmhouse during the school year, but of course we came home to live there every summer. Shirley's dad remodeled the farmhouse, and made a nice apartment on the back of the house out of the summer kitchen and woodshed.

For my last year at school we rented a third floor apartment on Stewart Avenue, above the Red & White grocery store. Shirley had never seen a cockroach before. When we moved in that fall, the roaches were so bad that the napkins were moving on the table! We had to fumigate the place before we could settle back in. We'll never forget when there was a fire downstairs in the grocery store. We never found out how the fire started, but we were sure thankful that our family got out safely. Our friend and boarder, Scoop Lewis, grabbed Diane, and I got Linda out of the house in time. Luckily, there was very little damage to our place.

Our girls had been back and forth to campus in the car so many times, they could've made the trip blindfolded. One day Shirley was frantic when they turned up missing—Diane was seven years old and Linda was only four at the time. They had found a stray dog where they were playing and brought it to the clinic on campus, about a half mile away, so I could fix it up.

GRADUATION, 1950

We didn't see much of Dean Hagan until we graduated. He came back from Europe and Plum Island a few times during the course of our studies and was there to hand out the diplomas.

I took the State Boards at Cornell the week before graduation. They weren't too difficult because we were well-prepared and ready, and I got my diploma. Shirley and the girls were there to watch me graduate, and my four sisters came out for the event. I was proud that day of all we had accomplished together.

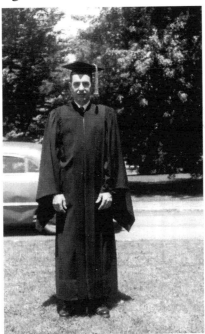

Dr. Stanley E. Garrison

The day after graduation, the Dean's secretary called. I was in the shower when the call came, and Shirley took the message that Dr. Hagan wanted me to stop in and see him. To have the Dean request for someone to come in was pretty special, because he had hardly known any of us through the years we were there. We were getting ready to return to Burnt Hills, the kids were packing their dolls and Shirley was boxing up our things—we couldn't get out of there fast enough. I remember getting dressed and putting on a good suit and tie. Normally I didn't get dressed up to go down to the college. It was more likely that I would wear coveralls and boots! I'm not exactly sure what Shirley said to me, but I know that her fear was that the Dean was going to talk me into staying.

When I arrived on campus I asked the secretary what I was in for, but she just instructed me to tap on the door and go on in. Once inside, Dean Hagan put a hand on my shoulder and said, "Dr Garrison, take a seat, I've got something to tell you." He told me that there was an opening at the college for an intern, and asked if I'd be interested. I hated to tell him that what I wanted most was to go home, so I made a compromise, and said that I'd be glad to stay for the summer, until the next class came in September. He was very happy, and said that it would fill in the void while some of the professors took their vacations. Shirley took the news well. She was glad to learn that I'd be working four 10-hour days and would be able to come home to Burnt Hills to be with her and the girls on the weekends. By staying on and working in the small animal clinic for the summer, I really learned a lot of things. Dr. Ellis Leonard, head of the clinic, was a helpful mentor.

It was during that summer that Dr. Hagan asked me to go with him to the Rotary Club meeting and luncheon at the hotel downtown. It was quite an experience. I had no idea what a Rotary Club did, but after that luncheon I started thinking about starting a Rotary club in Burnt Hills when I got home. I felt that Rotary was a good organization to get involved in because the local business and professional leaders worked together to help their own communities as well as people around the world.

Dean Hagan also asked me if I knew any of the legislators in Albany. The college needed funding to either repair the lab and other old facilities or to build a new veterinary complex on the hill east of the campus. I told him that one of the oldest Senators in Albany, Gilbert T. Seelye, was my neighbor. The Senator owned 200 acres in Burnt Hills. I knew him well enough, and we had even combined his oats for him once. I arranged a meeting with Senator Seelye, and the Dean and I were both pleased by the outcome. The veterinary college's needs were considered for funding, and it was a beginning to promote the double benefit of researching some diseases that affected people as well as animals.

THE FIRST BURNT HILLS
VETERINARY HOSPITAL

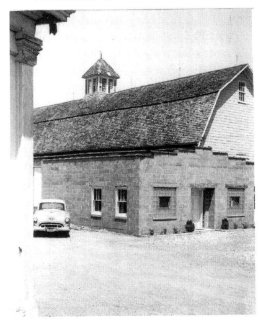

1950

After finishing the renovations on our farmhouse in Burnt Hills, Shirley's dad, Harris Miller, also remodeled the ice house and milk room at the farm, and put on an addition, making us a modern little veterinary hospital. Mr. Miller was retired and looked forward to the work. He was a great carpenter and it was a beautiful setup. The front part of the building was a comfortable animal clinic, with seats along the wall in the waiting room, and an observation window that allowed people to see their pets as they recovered. It was just like watching a new baby in a maternity ward! In fact, the light in the surgery room came from the hospital in Amsterdam. The back part of the hospital was the large animal clinic where we did many caesareans and rumenotomies ("hardware" operations to remove nails or fence staples swallowed by ruminant animals–usually cows–which could pierce through the stomach wall and into the heart). It had a big box stall where animals could stay overnight. All of that floor space was heated, and we were tickled to have a nice place to work.

When we started out, the business was 70% large animal cases, and 30% small animal. Shirley will tell you, we worried about how many calls we'd need in order to make a go of it! When we hung out the shingle which read, "Burnt Hills Veterinary Hospital," over the door of the clinic in the fall of 1950, we thought we'd need to make three calls a day, at six dollars a call. We figured that on $18 a day we could make it just fine! We laugh about that small amount now, but it was serious business at that time.

THE MILLERS

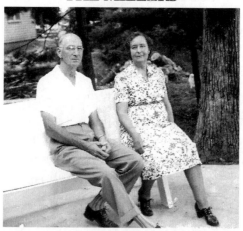

Harris and Ethel Miller

When Shirley's folks, Harris and Ethel, came into the picture, it was like having a second set of parents. We wouldn't have been nearly as successful without them! They were special people, and had been through some hard times of their own.

Mr. Miller was a great carpenter, and business was going well until the Depression hit. He took a job with a construction company, and had to move from place to place following the work. The family spent a lot of time in the Adirondacks where Mr. Miller helped build the Plattsburgh Normal School (now Plattsburgh State University) and the Tuberculin Sanitarium in Raybrook. There wasn't much money to rent or buy a place, so they camped in their tent for a couple of summers. Shirley and her brother Erwin, who was five years older, remember those years as being a lot of fun. They spent their time hunting, fishing and enjoying the outdoors.

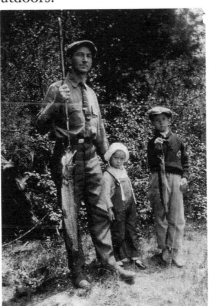

Harris, Shirley and Erwin Miller going fishin'

Shirley's dad was at the point of retiring when he and Ethel came to live at the farm, and we needed a lot of things done! Her dad was glad to have the work and help us out. Mr. Miller kept a diary, and may have only written a total of four or five sentences a day but he kept track of everything. Shirley's folks didn't have much money or a lot of needs and together were kind of like bread and jam—they came out pretty even.

PRACTICING IN THE 50'S
A FAMILY BUSINESS

By the time our little vet hospital opened, Burnt Hills had a population of 4,000–doubling what it had been fifty years earlier.

I was able to split my time between my work. There were some days when I was farming, and others when I was practicing veterinary medicine. I can remember people with concerns about their animals coming to get me while I was working in the fields. I'd quit what I was doing and take a look. It never really bothered me to switch between the two at a moments notice. I enjoyed doing both as my grandson, Mike, remembers me singing that familiar song, ..."Whatever will be, will be." Maybe some of my classmates from Cornell might have frowned on it, saying to choose one career or the other, but we did what we needed to do.

Burnt Hills was a very small village, but we'd set up our hospital in a progressive area where we really just couldn't miss. There were new houses and new people arriving all the time. General Electric was booming, and Burnt Hills became a bedroom community. The place grew right around us, and it wasn't long before we had more work than we could handle.

When the hospital first opened, Shirley and I did everything ourselves. Shirley took care of the animals, assisted me with surgery, answered the phone, and did the bookwork as well as all the cleaning. Diane and Linda did what they could in the office and even helped clean up after surgeries. We had a family business, all right!

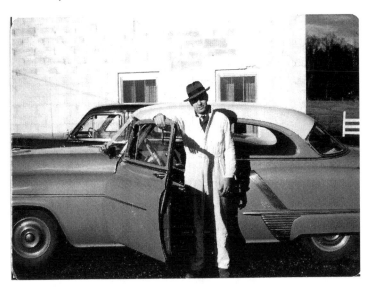

Doc & the Practice Car

In April of 1953 our third daughter, Laurie, was born. Things were getting busier at the hospital, and with the new baby, there was more than enough for Shirley to do. We were just realizing that we needed some help when help found us! Rachel Hubbel came to us just out of high school. She had a horse that was lame, so we treated it, and she kept the horse at the farm. She hung around at the hospital a bit wanting to work. We definitely needed the help so she became our first hospital employee. Rachel was the kind of girl who could do anything and everything. She cleaned the hospital, fed heifers, mowed the lawn, helped put in hay–a real all around gal. Her mother and father were quite old, and she became like a daughter to us. One of her classmates says to this day that Rachel was one of the best athletes that Burnt Hills ever had. Our family was devastated when several years later we lost our dear friend, Rachel, to breast cancer.

While they helped care for other peoples' animals, our daughters raised their own as well. Diane and Laurie had horses, and Linda liked the cows. We named our farm Laur-Lin-Dee Farm after the girls, and they helped with the chores and loved to go with me on calls.

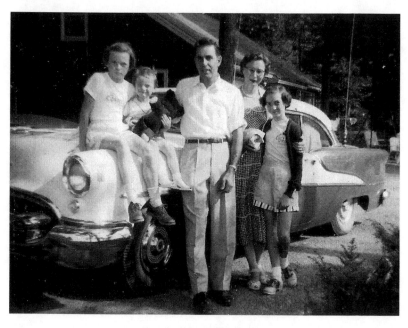

Our family, mid-1950's

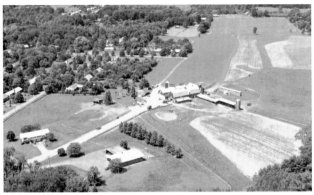

Aerial of Home Farm, Duplex and Veterinary Hospital in foreground

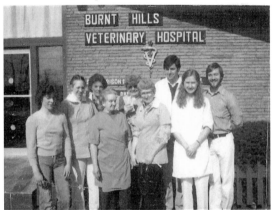

Burnt Hills Veterinary Hospital Staff - 1983
(L-R) Kathy Sisler, Lyn Mackerer, Pat Pustolka, Frances Heath,
Jean Carr, Ann Yager, Dr. Michael Rach, Dr. Laurie Ellis,
& Dr. Peter Farrell

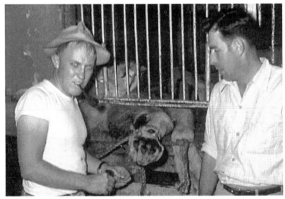

Circus Lion - 1957 Gordon Layton, veterinary student, (at left)
and Dr. Stan Garrison setting a lion's broken leg

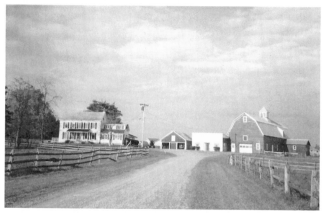

Garrison Home Farm on Goode Street in Burnt Hills, circa 1965

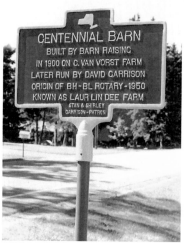

Historical Marker erected in 2000 at 145 Goode Street

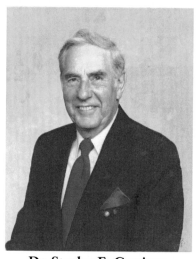

Dr. Stanley E. Garrison
1986 -87 Rotary District 7190 Governor

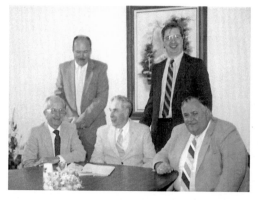

BH-BL Rotary Committee 1986-1987
(L-R) Alfred Fritz, Charles McLoughlin, Stan Garrison, Robert VanVranken & Terry Morris

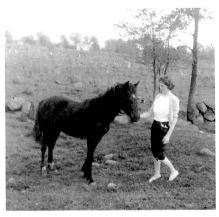

Diane
and foal, Echo
1960

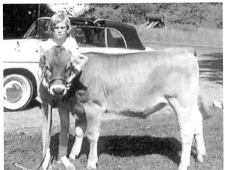

Linda
and Brown Swiss heifer, "Linda"

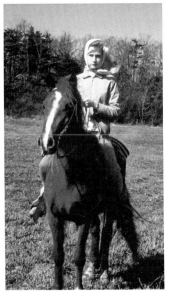

Laurie
and "Cherokee"

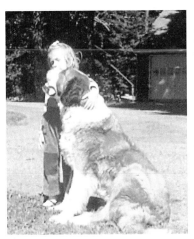

Peppy, St. Bernard
bigger than Laurie,
constant companion to our three girls

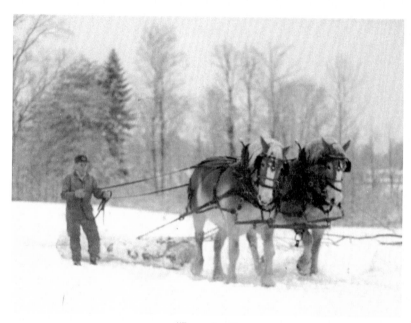

"Logging"
Stan driving team, skidding logs out of our woods

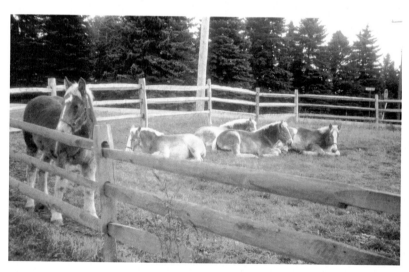

Five Belgian Fillies
born at our home farm 1981

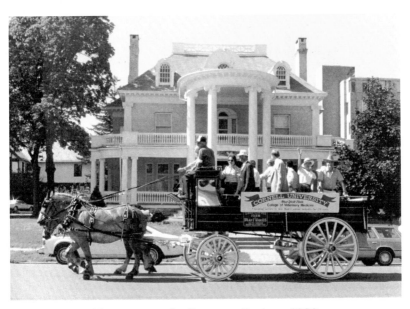

Travers parade, Saratoga Springs 1990
Stan's Show Wagon and team of Belgians for
Cornell University College of Veterinary Medicine

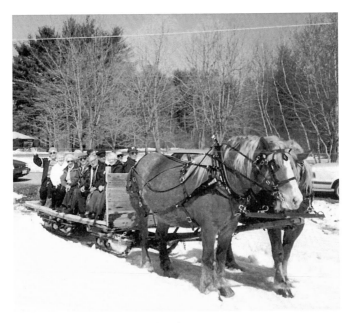

Sleighride in 1990
BH-BL Golden Grads, 1934-1937

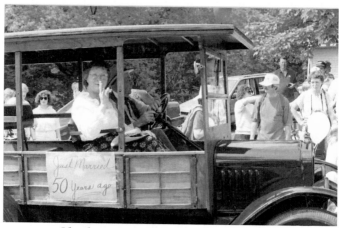

Charlton Founder's Day Parade 1992
Shirley & Stan in their 1924 Model-T Ford Depot Hack

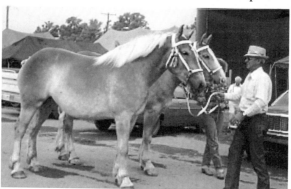

"Honey and Easter"
Belgian mares with Robert Anderson

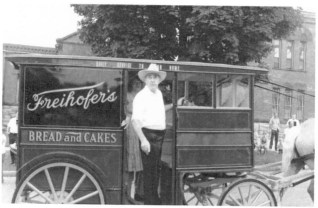

Freihofer Wagon
Stan, Linda Driving

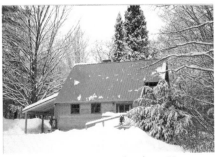

Cabin at Stratford, N.Y.

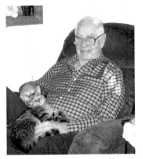

Stan & "Jenna"
Enjoying retirement

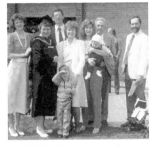

**Shirley's graduation
in 1987 from
Fulton-Montgomery
Community College**
(L-R) Granddaughter
Amy, Shirley,
Grandson Mike,
Linda, Laurie, Stan,
Jay Walter,
Grandsons
Matthew and Derek

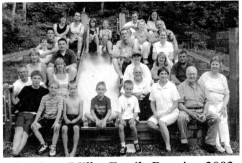

Garrison/Miller Family Reunion 2002

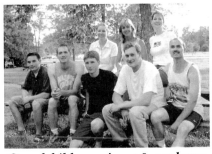

Grandchildren, nieces & nephews
(L-R) Matthew, Michael, Derek, Darlene,
Lynne, Nathan, Amy, Jeffrey

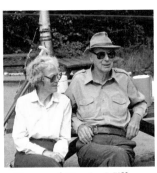

Dot and Erwin Miller
(Shirley's brother and
sister-in-law)
50th Anniversary 1988

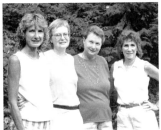

Laurie, Linda, Shirley & Diane

Burnt Hills Veterinary Hospital

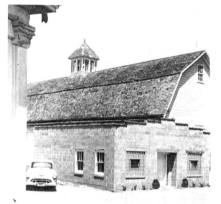

1950

1961

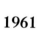
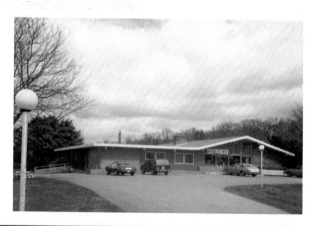

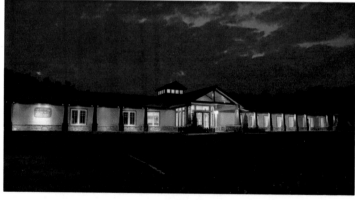

2005

VETERINARY TAILS

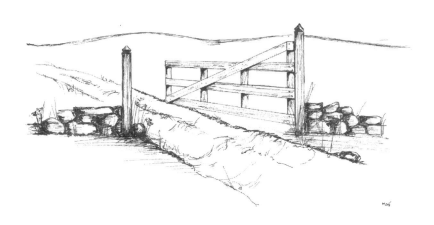

INTRODUCTION TO VETERINARY STORIES

There are so many memorable veterinary stories that have occurred over the years—not to mention a lot of good help from a number of associates who worked with us—far too many to record them all.

We all understood that treatment of an animal meant treatment of the owner as well. When a farmer called we knew we were dealing with valuable animals that brought him his livelihood. Pets were equally important, though for different reasons. A couple with no children could become frantic when their companion dog was injured and in need of immediate attention. Treating both large and small animals brought us into contact with a variety of situations.

Most cases were pretty straightforward, but sometimes I could hear myself saying, "This is no Boy Scout project!" In every case, I had to be able to make decisions—sometimes instantly, and maybe it wasn't always the right one, but I couldn't wait too long to do it.

Over the years, the anatomy part didn't change, but the pharmaceuticals changed dramatically, and as new veterinarians entered the practice, we were able to learn from each other. Occasionally, I was able to show young graduates a procedure they had never seen before, and would tell them, "Boys, that's not on page 99."

We were satisfied with the outcome of our cases almost every time, and I've always said that we couldn't have done any better, in business or in life.

PEPPY

It seems that the most appropriate story to start with is how we came to have our first real family pet. While working at Cornell in the small animal clinic the summer after graduation, a man called to say that his St. Bernard was having trouble trying to deliver her puppies. She had already given birth to twelve pups at home and laid on four of them. When he brought her in, she was unconscious due to a condition called Eclampsia (hypocalcemia). We began giving her calcium intravenously, and she started to come around. After she awoke fully, she delivered two more healthy puppies.

The next morning when the man came to pick up the dog, he said he'd give me a pup, so I picked one out. I chose a nice female, and brought her home when she was weaned. The girls named our puppy "Peppy," and boy did she grow fast! One day we had to take the bathtub out because she got stuck behind it. All the neighbors loved her, and she greeted everybody with her big tail going around in circles. Peppy was a loyal pet, and even starred in a play that required three St. Bernard dogs. She was always available at the vet hospital, and eventually became a real rescue dog when she provided blood for transfusions for several dogs. One client was so happy that we were able to save her dog through a transfusion that she brought Peppy a big bone tied with a red bow for Christmas.

MILK FEVER

One of my first large animal calls was for a case of Milk Fever in a small Guernsey herd. Milk Fever is a funny thing—it's caused by a calcium deficiency at calving, and cows can react differently to treatment. It's a fairly common condition, but one that could easily kill a cow as well. The farmer had already had one veterinarian treat this cow, but she was still in pretty bad shape. A big butcher knife was hanging over a tenon in the barn, and the farmer nodded at that and snarled, "Boy, if that cleaver was there when that other vet was here, I'd have had meat!" I started to work on the cow, cutting the dose of calcium, and giving it real slow. When the cow started groaning, I glanced at that knife—I wasn't sure if the farmer was going to use it on me! The cow pulled through in the end, but could have gone the other way. I had a cow die once just like that. I didn't blame the other veterinarian either since symptoms don't always present themselves consistently. It's really a matter of being there at the right time.

Another case of Milk Fever occurred quite late in the day, office hours had ended, and a woman called us from several miles away. I had never been to her farm before, but she said that her cow had been having trouble calving all afternoon. Her veterinarian had been there for two hours and still hadn't been able to get the calf out. Her vet had called the cattle dealer to come and get the cow to sell it for beef, which seemed to be the only option. The woman said she just wanted me to take another look.

It was a difficult situation, and by the time I got there the cattle dealer was sitting on a milk stool in the feed room, waiting to see what would happen. The cow that was down was a Guernsey, and the woman cared for these cattle while her husband worked in a mill. She had four girls running back and forth to the house for whatever was needed—towels, water, soap. They just wanted to help.

I knew very well that the vet who had been there before me had worked on this cow for a long time, and I don't blame him for giving up. She had not shown any dilation of the cervix, so I tapped on her eye to check her reflexes—there was no response. I suspected she was coming down with Milk Fever. Usually a cow doesn't show signs of the illness until after calving, but it can work different ways. Again, I happened to be there at the right time, and had the advantage of seeing this animal several hours later than the previous veterinarian.

I started a slow drip of calcium gluconate, and gave her two bottles over a long period. Pretty soon she started to wink a little bit, teardrops came to her eyes, and her milk began to drip. You should have heard that cattle dealer who was waiting to take her away, "You son of a gun, that cow's gonna get up." She rose up enough to lift her head, and then started to dilate. Everything seemed to come to life, and we delivered a live heifer calf.

The owner of the cow gave me a big hug, and her four daughters were smiling from ear to ear. These people were tickled that I had been able to save their cow and her calf. I always say, "the person who sees the animal last has the advantage of the most information, and the best chance to save it."

The most unusual case involving Milk Fever I ever encountered though occurred about eight or ten miles from our place. The call came in late, about 9:00 at night, from a family that had just one cow. The man said, "I've got a Jersey cow that's going to die. She had a calf yesterday, and the calf seems fine, but the cow can't get up." Right away I knew it was Milk Fever, and explained that the cow was going to need some medicine. The man was quick to ask, "Well, could you come tonight? If you don't, she'll be dead in the morning."

Shirley said she'd go with me, and when we arrived it was just as I had suspected. As with the other cases, we gave the cow a bottle of calcium, but Jersey cows tend to respond quickly. There was nothing unusual about it, but as the calcium kicked in the cow was still shivering, and I told the owner that we'd stay for a bit to see how she made out.

While she was recovering, the man said, "Why don't you come on up to the house and have some cake. It's my daughter's birthday. She's seven years old and her grandma just sent her an alligator and a watermelon from Florida." He took us inside and showed us—and sure enough, there was an alligator, about two feet long, floating in the bathtub with the watermelon! I don't know what they were going to do with that alligator.

TEPP (1957)

One of our most serious cases happened just up the road from the hospital and involved my own cattle. My neighbor, who had an orchard and dairy farm, had sold his cows and offered me the use of his pasture for my heifers. I turned out 14 Holstein heifers to be bred with my Black Angus bull.

When it was time to do pregnancy checks, Shirley's dad and Gordon, our junior student from Cornell, came with me to help move the cattle across the road into my neighbor's old barn. It was mid-afternoon on a very hot July day. We took a pail of grain to entice them into the barn and into their stanchions. If all of the heifers were bred, we were going to remove the bull.

I confirmed that all 14 cows were pregnant, so we set to work moving the bull. I remember just getting ahold of his halter when he jerked back, and pulled out two of the wooden stanchions. The bull, as well as the heifer next to him got loose, and ran into the barnyard. When the animals ran back into the barn, they came in through a different door, one that had old fruit boxes and spray material piled around it. The bull was the first in. He had just gotten through the opening when he dropped dead on the floor. The heifer was right behind him and dropped in a matter of seconds—both of them were dead.

We smelled a chemical odor, very penetrating to the nose, so we closed the door and went to see the neighbor who owned an apple orchard. I asked the neighbor if he knew of any spray material stored next door in the barn. He said that there might be as he had previously bought some TEPP from the farmer. Tetra-ethyl-pyrophosphate was a spray material used on pears and he had a spray mask that stated, "not good for TEPP". He suggested that we call the State Troopers to investigate because he had seen little children playing in the barn. He also said that we should notify Cornell University Poison Control to advise us what to do.

Someone did come from Cornell the next day, and with the State Troopers, confirmed that it was indeed TEPP that had killed the animals. The bull and heifer had stepped on an old can of TEPP that was being stored in that barn. The chemical penetrated through the hide, and killed the bull and heifer instantly—a deadly case of phosphate poisoning. It's scary to think about it, but kids in the neighborhood would often play hide-and-seek around that barn on the weekends. We lost two animals, but we may have saved some human lives, and thank goodness my father-in-law, Gordon, and I had not stepped on that can too. That day, the Troopers found seven cans of TEPP in the old hay where the children had played.

SHEEP CAN BE SCARED TO DEATH

A few times we were called when a pack of dogs had killed some sheep. When that happened, I would have to assess the value of the sheep, so the farmer could get paid for his loss by the State. I would always tell people when they called, "Don't be in too much of a hurry for me to get there. If you've got six dead sheep today, you may have eight by tomorrow. Sometimes a few more die from pure fright!" It sounds impossible, but it's true—sheep get so nervous.

On one of these calls, I went to the house and rapped on the door, but no one was around. I figured that the family was all out with the sheep, but when I looked down, standing there was the cutest little Korean girl who was just beginning to talk. She was on the other side of the screen, stark naked. She said in her small voice, "There's nobody home." I assumed that she had probably just woken from a nap or something, but that's all she could say. I told her, "Okay, honey, we'll find somebody," and I picked her up and carried her down to the barn to her folks. They did lose a few more sheep from fright that day.

Sometimes you run into the funniest things. I just wonder where that little girl is today.

SIMPLE DETECTIVE WORK

Early one January morning, during some bitter cold weather, a man called the hospital and said that he wanted me to come right away. He sounded very agitated and said that some dogs had been at his place in the night and killed his best cow. I said, "If the cow is dead, there's no big hurry is there?" He said, "Oh yes, I've got to collect on her, the Town Board's got a meeting tonight." The man claimed that the dogs had ripped the ear on his old Jersey cow, and chewed her tail during the attack.

I went down to inspect the animal, and knew right away he was pulling my leg. For one thing, he was too anxious to get his money, and secondly, the damaging marks appeared to have come from a knife. One of the cow's ears was badly severed, so I offered, "I'll cut this ear off and give it to the assessors."

When I brought the ear to the town officials, they were having a heated discussion. One of them made the comment, "That's the trouble with dogs running loose. They ought to be shot." Another one turned to me and asked, "What do you think happened here?" I showed them the ear, and where a sharp knife had cut it from the outside going in. I explained that a dog would bite the ear and pull out on it the other way. It was very simple detective work. The town official remarked, "Gee, that's right—I didn't think of that," and they refused to pay the claim.

I believe that in this case, the old cow just died. The cold weather may have finished her off, and the man thought he could get some money for his loss.

SHORT OF MILK

A farmer called one night, and asked me to come to his farm the next morning. He was going out of business, and getting ready to sell his cows. "I've been short of milk for the last three or four days," he said, "and I can't figure out what's wrong." The farmer had a fairly new pipeline, and had also just replaced his vacuum pump. "I've spent a lot of money here already, and have to get these cows back in shape and milking well for the sale," he explained. I told him that I would be down in the morning, and not to turn the cows out, sweep the barn, or start the gutter cleaner before I got there. I wanted to be able to inspect the surroundings before anything was disturbed.

When I got to his place, a group of neighboring farmers had gathered to try and resolve this mystery—all the pickups were there. I went into the milkroom, set my case down, and turned on the faucets in the washtubs. A shortage of milk usually has something to do with the water—you can feed a cow all you want, but if she doesn't get water, you don't get milk. There was plenty of pressure in the milkroom, so I shut off the water, stepped down on the landing, and inside the barn. The first cow in the row—of about 40 in all—was a big Brown Swiss. She was kind of thick over the shoulders like a beef cow and had blood on the back of her tail. I walked down behind the cattle, looked in the drop, and paused near the bull on the end.

Leaning against the back wall of the barn the farmers had formed a line, glancing at the cows and discussing the problem. I commented, "You fellas have been here a while," and asked them, "What do you think is wrong?" We all knew each other, so one of them shot back with a grin, "You're the veterinarian, you tell us!" I said, "Give me a minute to finish my inspection and I'll let you know."

This time I walked in front of the cows. I could see that they still had plenty of hay and silage to eat as I approached that first big Brown Swiss. When I got closer to her head, I noticed a change in odor—it was a strong, sweet smell. I pushed on the lever in her water bowl, which made a hissing noise, and only a trickle came out. She looked at the bowl, and the other cows turned their heads our way, like they wanted a drink too.

I turned to the farmers and said, "Well, I think I know what the trouble is." When I had looked in the gutter I saw that the manure behind those cows was dry like the bull's—in kind of a curl—which means that none of them were getting enough water. I could see that the big Brown Swiss had calved recently, and still had some blood on her tail. By the amount of fat she carried, this cow had probably been dry a long time. When the fatty tissue builds up, the liver throws off acetic acid, which I could smell on her breath. The condition is called Acetonemia. There's a nervous kind and a dumb kind. This cow had an acute case, and acted nervous. She had been sucking on the soft copper pipe next to her and squeezed it flat, so water couldn't come through the pipe to the rest of the herd from the milkroom.

I treated the cow, but told the farmer he'd have to get a plumber to fix the pipe!

RABIES

In 1957 we had a new assistant county agricultural agent who hadn't seen the southern end of our county, and asked if he could ride with me on some calls. One morning in May, he met me at the hospital, and a call came in from that area. The farmer said, "I've been feeding potatoes to my cows, and I think one has a potato stuck in her throat."

So the county agent went with me to investigate. The farmer had cleaned out the storage in his cellar, and the bags of potatoes were lined up in the barn in front of the feed room. The rest of the cows were turned out in the barnyard, so it was easy to observe our patient. This cow's behavior was quite unusual—she was moving back and forth in her stall, and pulling back quick on the stanchion. She also slobbered at the mouth, had profuse diarrhea, and her eyes were glazed.

The county agent was scared that the cow was rabid, and I was too, so right away I encouraged him to stay back. I said to the farmer, "I hope you haven't had your arm down her throat," and he said he hadn't.... "Well, not all the way—I had a ball bat and was trying to work at that potato." As we stood there, the cow broke out of the wooden stanchion, jumped through an empty silo door, and expired right there.

I asked the farmer if he had seen any rabid animals near his cows. He remembered that one of his employees had seen a fox in the barn—but that had been back in the fall. What the farmer didn't know was that the incubation period for rabies is pretty long; it can take months for a bite below the hock to reach the brain.

After putting rubber gloves on, I went into the silo to remove the cow's head and placed it in a garbage can. We called in a report, and the Troopers came to take our specimen to the lab. It wasn't long before the lab confirmed the cow was rabid. A doctor at the lab advised everyone who had been exposed to the cow to take a series of shots. He said, "We'll send you 14 vials of the vaccine—if you don't take them all, you might as well not take any."

I first went to my doctor, who gave me four of the shots, in alternating arms. When I started to get a pink streak under one arm, he refused to give me any more. I went to another doctor, who understood his colleague's hesitation, but said he'd give me four more. That made eight, and I had six shots left. I figured that if I was going to die anyway, I was going to take them all.

Shirley and I were looking to buy an Elkhound dog at the time, and located one in northern Vermont. We packed up the syringes and needles, and the rest of the vaccine. I decided I would give the remaining shots to myself. On the way to pick up the Elkhound, we stopped to see a friend who had worked with me at G.E. He was a big fella who did a lot of butchering, and his wife was a rugged Canadian. We boiled the needles on their stove, and I drew up the vaccine in the syringe to take the shot. The next thing we knew, our big butcher friend had passed out and hit his head on the floor.

We had a lot of clients like that at the vet hospital—the bigger they were, the harder they'd fall. They'd talk about blood and guts, or what they'd seen in the war, but as soon as you'd look in their kitten's ears, they'd pass out. You could almost pick 'em.

I managed to finish taking the series of rabies shots and, as they say, lived to tell about it.

POISON

A call came in early one Monday morning about a horse that was seriously ill. It was an older mare that was so weak she could barely stand. The owner said that a veterinarian from the racetrack had been there on Sunday, but could not determine what was wrong.

I looked at the horse, and she was pathetic, bracing herself in the doorway of the barn. Her neck was arched, and her eyes were closed in pain. I lifted her lips, and her membranes were so light colored that I suspected some kind of poisoning. I looked around for a possible source of the poison, but found nothing. I learned that a pony shared the pasture with the horse, but had none of these symptoms, and appeared in perfect health.

The owner and her family thought the world of this mare, and couldn't imagine what it had gotten into. At the same time, she didn't want the horse to continue suffering in this state if there was no cure.

I drew a vial of blood and brought the sample back to the hospital to check her hemoglobin level. It was as low as it could possibly be—her red blood cells were completely ruptured or lyced (hemolytic anemia), which indicated poisoning. The owner wanted to know the truth, and I told her that the mare should be put down. The family agreed, and called a man with a backhoe to bury their old friend. This was not how I liked to see a case turn out, but it was the most humane treatment.

After I put the horse to sleep, I was still bothered that we hadn't found the cause. I walked the fence line of the pasture, and saw nothing unusual. A storm had broken the limb of a red maple tree, and it was hanging over the fence, into the pasture. The leaves on the dying limb were dried, and when I got closer, I noticed where some had been stripped off and most likely eaten by the horse.

I took some of the leaves with me, and sent them to Cornell to be tested. No one at the college had ever heard of a case of poisoning from red maple leaves, but it was similar to the toxins in Sudan grass during a dry year (prussic acid poisoning). Under certain conditions, plants can build up a substance that converts to prussic acid—a rapidly acting poison that travels through the bloodstream, preventing the cells from using oxygen. With more investigation, the Cornell veterinarians discovered that this had been seen before with red maple leaves in England, but was the first case to be documented here. Apparently, under certain conditions, there is something about red maple leaves that horses like.

I wondered why the pony had not been affected, and figured that the branch may have been too high to reach, or the horse may have chased him away. This experience taught me to consider even the most ordinary things when analyzing a case.

HORSE IN THE POOL

There's a dairy farmer and humorist in our county who wrote a book about a cow in the pool, and it really did happen—twice on his farm! Well, I had the experience of rescuing a horse from a pool! This was in a high-class neighborhood, back in the days when very few people had their own swimming pools.

It was a day in January, and a client's horse had gotten loose from the barn. We had a few inches of snow on the ground, and the animal wandered toward the house, and onto the cover of their in-ground pool. The horse broke through the pool cover and the layer of ice on the water, and was struggling to get out. We had to think quickly with that horse in the frigid water, so we called in a tow truck, and fashioned a ramp from some building materials. After a few attempts, we were able to get the horse's feet on the platform, and steady him enough so he could walk out of the water.

Usually it's the people who need to watch where they walk around animals; this time it was the other way around.

CIRCUS LION

In 1957 a man who owned a traveling circus called to ask if we would take a look at a male lion. The animal had broken his rear leg in a motorcycle accident while trick-riding with a female lion inside a wooden silo. I suspected it was one of my classmates from veterinary college just having fun.

I listened to the gentleman on the phone who said he could not get any veterinarian to even look at the lion. He indicated that the accident had happened five days before, and the lion was becoming weak and refusing to eat. I thought the words "refusing to eat" were the best news yet.

The circus, called "Stratt's Show," was stationed in Fort Edward, New York, north of Saratoga Springs and was due to move out the next day to Schenectady. They were going to set up on what was called Hungry Hill, where those events usually took place. I told the owner that we had never worked on a lion, but that we would look at him the following day when the circus arrived in Schenectady. He was relieved to have finally secured a veterinarian who would examine the lion, and if nothing could be done, would have the ability to euthanize the big cat.

The circus owner called the next day around noontime and indicated that they had unloaded and placed the lion cage under a tree to allow some relief from the extreme heat. My father-in-law, along with Gordon, a junior student from Cornell, and I drove down to the circus thinking we may be on a goose chase, but went prepared to do what we could. We took the x-ray machine, leadropes to restrain the animal, anesthesia for I.V. if needed, and "Dad" had his camera to take pictures of all our maneuvers.

This was a huge lion weighing 550 pounds, according to George, the caretaker. He had not eaten for the last two days, but seemed strong enough when we attempted to restrain him! We decided to give I.V. anesthesia in one foreleg and tied the other foreleg with a rope running outside of the cage anchored to a circus truck. Although we cut the dose to half, the amount (per pound of weight) of what was recommended for a domestic cat, this fellow ended up sleeping for five days!

With the lion safely slumbering, we took an x-ray of the leg and then put an 8-inch threaded steel rod through the broken stub. When we were satisfied with the placement, we took another x-ray just to confirm that the leg would work fine. All of our work in pinning this lion's leg had to be secured under the skin. George, the caretaker, told us that a lion would not tolerate a bandage and would chew his own leg off in order to remove the dressing.

This lion did recover and we received a card from the circus' winter quarters in Florida saying that the owner was pleased with the surgery. He also indicated that he would call when the circus returned the next summer to give us a report on the lion and have us check his progress. Word of our "expertise" with exotic animals must have gotten around. One day we ended up working on a camel with a broken jaw that was more difficult to handle than the lion!

OLD STALLION

We had this one client who didn't call very often, but when he did, it was an experience just getting into his barn. He had this big barn door that was just overwhelming to try to open; it was held to the doorframe with pieces of leather for hinges. The funny thing was, this old fella had worked in a hardware store most of his life—he could have brought home anything he needed to fix that door!

I was called to his place to see an older stallion that had belonged to his wife; she had passed away some time ago, and this was the only animal he had left in the barn. He explained, "The horse won't eat anymore, and he keeps pulling back in the stall." It smelled bad in the dark barn that was loaded with cobwebs, and I spotted the stallion who was stamping his feet in the stall. I suspected a foot problem, and thought he might have stepped on a nail or something of that nature. I went into the stall and the horse leaned back, pulling his rope tight. The man went up ahead of the horse, cut the rope, and the stallion fell backwards, passing out right there. He was that bad when I saw him.

We couldn't find anything wrong with his feet, but he had this big halter on his head that the man had made out of a tractor belt. We got a flashlight, checked all around the stall, and discovered a big spike poking down through the ceiling. The stallion must have raised up in the stall and that nail poked through the halter, causing an abscess. There was no way for the abscess to drain in that position, and the horse had come down with tetanus.

There was nothing we could do for his stallion, but this gentleman lived to be 100 years old!

FIVE DEAD COWS

A good friend of mine had a small herd of Brown Swiss cattle. He called one day saying that he had found five of his cows dead when he'd gone to the barn early that morning. He had opened up a new bag of grain, and was sure that the deaths had something to do with the feed. He asked me to come and see what had poisoned these cattle.

We walked inside the milkroom, and he threw the switch on for the lights. As soon as he did that, I could see a horse through the open door of the barn doing the jitters, dancing around in his box stall. I said, "Shut off the juice—there's something wrong here electrically." When he shut off the switch, the horse calmed right down. There was probably wet bedding in the stall, and because of the size of their feet, horses absorb a shock more quickly.

With the power off, we walked through the barn with a flashlight, and he showed me the five dead cows in different locations. All of the cows had eaten the same feed, so I asked him what else he had done the day before, besides his normal routine chores. He thought a minute and said, "Well, it was so cold yesterday I stayed inside and worked on my water pump. I took the pipe out of the well that was rusted, and put in 16 feet of new inch-and-a-half plastic with a new foot-valve." That was the answer right there—the new plastic pipe that he had installed to replace the rusty pipe did not properly ground the pump, and the cows had been electrocuted when they drank from their metal water bowls.

MYNA BIRD

Two women who were clients from the city (Schenectady) had given us a myna bird, thinking a veterinarian might like such a unique bird. Although he was a gift, sometimes he was a real pain in the neck! People sitting in the waiting room could hear him talking, and he sounded just like a person: "Do you want to take a bath?" "What are you doing?" "How about that!" A client once came in to pick up some pills, and when she rang the bell at the desk, the myna bird said, "Go to hell."

One cold night, a woman called after 11:00 p.m., frantic about her cat that was badly hurt. We weren't at the hospital at that hour, but I told her to bring the cat in and I'd meet her there. I got to the clinic, unlocked the door, and turned a light on. I was getting some things ready in the back, when the lady came in with her cat wrapped in a towel—she was covered in blood. I heard that damn myna bird say to her, "Want to take a bath?" The poor woman was scared to death.

Once she had settled down a bit she told me what had happened. Apparently, her husband was supposed to pick up some milk for their baby and forgot. He had just come from work, so he decided to stay home with the baby while she went out for the milk. She started the car and didn't know that the cat had climbed up on the warm motor. When she backed out of the garage, the fan took the cat's ear and front leg off.

The woman's 7-year old daughter had come with her to the hospital in her nightgown and coat, and just knew that things were bad. I let her help me a little bit, and told her to put the cat on the heating pad. The cat was just about gone.

I said to the little girl, "I tell you what—if you go with me over to the big barn, we'll find you a kitten." I took the little girl by the hand and we all went to our barn, where she picked out the one she wanted. It made everything better for that little girl. We had two mother cats that kept producing kittens, and it was the best thing going. We often did that for families who lost a cat, and it seemed easier for them to handle their sorrow.

As for the myna bird, he got to be pretty well known in the area, and was even on the radio. Don Tuttle, from WGY radio, came up to the hospital one time and gave his "Farm Paper of the Air" report with the bird. I don't remember what the myna bird said while on the air, but thankfully it didn't need to be censored.

We were kind of sad when that myna bird finally expired, even though he was a noisy character!

BABE THE FREIHOFER'S HORSE

In the late 1950's Freihofer's was one of the last baking companies in the area to still peddle their bread and donuts with horse-drawn wagons. At that time, they had just a few routes left in Scotia and Schenectady, and these horses knew the streets better than the drivers! As the horses got older, and it became difficult to find drivers, the company phased out the wagon deliveries and transported everything by truck.

My daughter, Linda, once went with me to treat a sick delivery horse, and Bud Freihofer said she could have another one of their horses, Babe, a 21-year old Belgian. Babe was an old, quiet horse and he thought it would be good for Linda, who was eleven years old at the time, and nice for Babe to live out her days on our farm.

So Babe was given to Linda, along with a nice harness and wagon. A neighbor boy came with us to bring the horse home. Old Babe was ready when we got there, with plenty of oats in her nosebag. The horse was used to plodding along a certain route in Scotia, but Linda and Billy had to take her up Albany Street and over to Balltown Road in order to get home. They started out, and I followed behind in the car.

I had to stop along the way, long enough to re-check a client's horse, and Linda continued on ahead. She didn't get very far before a woman became suspicious and asked Linda, "Where are you going with that Freihofer wagon?" Linda explained that the horse and wagon were a gift from Mr. Freihofer, but the lady said, "Never on your life," and called the police. Linda was probably pushing on the lines to get Babe to go and running out of oats and time!

The officers came, and helped Linda get the horse and wagon to the police station. They put her in the police car and she told them, "My father has a two-way radio in his car too. Call him and he will tell you the horse belongs to me now." So Linda gave them the call number, KED735, and I answered and soon was at the police station to sort things out. She waited there while we brought two trucks to bring them home—one for the horse and one for the wagon.

Linda will never forget that day, her gift-horse Babe, and her run-in with the law.

GLUED TO THE TV

We had one client who would always wait until late at night to call us when he had an animal problem. Even if he knew he had trouble he'd wait to call because he had a new television, and wanted to watch his programs uninterrupted.

He was retired, not really a bona fide farmer, but he and his wife bought some Jerseys and a small farm, and that was what they wanted to do. It was a long way over to his place, and there were not many good roads on that route. When the snow was bad, it was especially difficult, and he was forever needing something done at that late hour! Whether it was a Milk Fever case or a prolapse, it didn't matter. He would call just like it was nine in the morning, and I was expected to be there.

When the man and his wife complained about the service we were providing, his wife said, "Let me come and work for you. I'll take the phone and make sure you get to the farms at the right time." We decided we'd hire her, and she worked one day, lasting only a few hours. "Oh God," she said, "I couldn't stand this." The couple was more understanding when they called us from then on.

THE FILLY AND DR. FOX

The first D.V.M. to work for us in 1958, Dr. Donald Fox, became like one of our family. He was raised on a farm and knew just how to adapt to large animal as well as small animal surgeries. Occasionally a farmer would have a calf, usually a purebred heifer, with an umbilical hernia. We were never sure whether the hernias resulted from the cow being clumsy and stepping on the calf's navel, or if it was hereditary. We never had more than one in any herd, but at the farms with registered cattle, it was worth the price for them to have us do the surgery and make a smooth repair. Apparently word got around about the bovine surgery and an owner of a four month old Thoroughbred from Saratoga Race Course asked if we could repair his filly's hernia.

During college we were not encouraged to do equine surgery as peritonitis would occur and the results were not satisfactory, but now that penicillin had been around a while, we said we would give it a try. Don and I sterilized a metal screen to place over the umbilical surgery site, and sewed it down making a stronger and safer repair. After finishing the surgery we were pleased with our results. The successful outcome brought our large animal hospital in Burnt Hills many calls from racehorse owners.

DR. DONALD FOX'S $400 SPAY

I remember a woman from the next county who owned a kennel, and raised boxer puppies. She suspected that one of her dogs might have a fallopian pregnancy, as she, herself, had once experienced.

She drove to our hospital in a big Buick with the boxer in the back. It was getting late when she came in, and we had just finished an umbilical hernia operation on a foal from the racetrack. My associate, Dr. Fox, was giving post-op instructions to the filly's owner when this woman took an interest in their conversation.

When they were finished, the lady asked the owner of the foal, "What does an operation like that cost?" He said, "I guess my bill was $400." This was a fairly sizeable figure at the time, and the first umbilical hernia surgery we had ever done on a filly.

So, before we even examined the woman's dog, she had a check all made out for $400 and gave it to Shirley! We did an exploratory surgery that night, discovered that her boxer was not pregnant, and spayed the dog at the woman's request. At that time a routine spay operation cost only about $23.

Dr. Fox had a lot of fun with this story, and when he went to the regional veterinary meeting, he asked the other vets, "What do you guys get for a spay these days?" and joked, "You better raise your prices, we just started charging $400!"

HEIFER CAESAREAN

As with our client who waited until late at night to call us, we also got our share of early morning calls. We once received a call at five one morning from a client who abruptly reported that one of his cows was down in the gutter. When he'd gone out to do his milking, he found the first-calf heifer had been trying to calve all night, and he thought he was going to lose her. Because she was in the gutter and couldn't get up, he was annoyed—he couldn't run the barn cleaner, and couldn't seem to work around her to milk the other cows. He had only a small herd of 20 cows, but he was in a hurry, and she was gumming up the works!

I gathered my instruments together, and brought along one of our technicians who lived next to us and who had agreed to give me a hand. We drove to the farm at that early hour, and found the heifer just as the owner had described—she couldn't move or get up. We rolled her over in the gutter onto clean straw, and tried to help her deliver. It was a big calf, and I couldn't reach the legs or find the head because it was folded back, So we decided to do a caesarean, which was very unusual on a cow. We did a nice operation by leadlight, and delivered a live heifer calf. I sewed the cow back up and when we were done, the client's first words were, "Do you think she'll give a pail of milk tonight?"

We were covered in blood and I almost felt like putting the calf back in! This was the way some people were—I'm sure that the man appreciated our saving the cow and calf; it just didn't come out that way.

Another call we had from this man involved a boxer puppy that his wife had given him for his birthday. The puppy had been vomiting, so I asked the man's wife if any small items were missing from around the house. She couldn't think of anything, so I opened up the puppy, and in its stomach found one of her silk stockings. I remember motioning to her husband to come see the ball of nylon, and he almost passed out. He was a big, burly guy.

This wasn't the first puppy to eat a stocking…or the last, but when women switched from stockings to pantyhose, we had fewer surgeries.

SNAKE BITE?

I was asked to examine a Pasofino mare that had been sent to Florida to be bred; she had marks on the skin of her jaw and was diagnosed with a rattlesnake bite. The owner was thoroughly upset to learn what had happened at the breeding ranch, and that such a thing could be fatal for both the mare and foal. It was suggested by the veterinary clinic in Florida that the mare be given antivenin (an antitoxin for venom produced by gradually increased injections of the snake venom).

I had some snake venom at the hospital, which we used for treating hot spots on nervous dogs. However, upon further examination with a mouth speculum, I found that the mare had a cracked tooth. Not wishing to give the mare venom, we decided to remove the cracked tooth first.

It turned out that the mare was not poisoned by a snake bite afterall. While grazing in Florida, she had been kicked in the jaw by another horse. The mare went on to have a beautiful foal, and was fine after that.

PROLAPSE

There used to be a lot of auctions on farms, and it was common for buyers to visit the farm beforehand to check the quality of the merchandise. I remember one such auction was coming up in the next town. A local farmer had visited the farm the night before the sale to milk a particular cow of interest. He was assured, "She's the best cow in the herd," so the next day he bought her for a hefty sum at the auction.

When he got the cow home, she had her calf and prolapsed, expelling her uterus. This farmer wasn't a regular client of ours, but he didn't want anyone to learn what had happened to his new, expensive cow. He was known for his shrewd business deals, and to have word leak out about this investment-turned-sour would have been too embarrassing.

A friend of mine, a fellow farmer, went with me on the call. He had never seen a prolapse before, and after that day, he hoped never to have it happen on his farm. I worked to get the cow's reproductive tract back in place, and she coughed, reversing the progress I had made. This happened several times, but we were eventually successful and able to save the cow. After observing my repeated attempts, my friend summed up the painstaking process: "That's like trying to put spaghetti back in a wildcat's ass." How we laughed! It was the best medicine for that frustrating experience, and there were thousands more just like it that we probably don't even remember.

SKUNK IN THE GARBAGE CAN

We had clients who truly lived up to their last name of Kidder—they were always joking around. The wife called one night saying that they had a skunk in their yard that looked suspicious and might have rabies. I told her to have her husband get a garbage can and lid ready, and I would be right over. I was on my way to a meeting at the time, so I arrived at their place dressed in a suit. Turns out the Kidders weren't kidding—there really was a skunk waddling around in a sort of stupor. It was a dumb thing to do, but I picked up the skunk by the tail and threw him in the garbage pail, lucky not to be sprayed, scratched or bitten. The skunk was tested and found to be rabid.

Soon after that incident, the couple called on a Sunday morning. The husband had fallen and hurt his wrist, and asked if I would take an x-ray. Mrs. Kidder came into the hospital, leading her husband, who had on a dog collar and was down on all fours. We had a good laugh with the Kidders that day. He really did need an x-ray but it turned out that the wrist wasn't broken.

CHARLIE THE CHIMPANZEE

I can tell you that chimpanzees are probably the worst animals to handle. They look at a person one way with their eyes, and their tails and feet go in the other direction. In my few experiences with them, they scared me to death.

A lady who lived a few towns away from us had a little circus and a chimpanzee named Charlie. He was a male chimp, who weighed about 30 pounds, and needed some teeth taken out. They were sharp, like the needle teeth on a baby pig, and we told the client they would grow back if we pulled them. She wanted them out anyway so Charlie couldn't nip anyone in the meantime.

We had a job getting him under anesthesia, so the lady pulled out a pack of her Old Gold cigarettes, tamped one out for Charlie, lit it, and gave it to him. She let him smoke it while she was talking outside. He was pretty smart already at his age (when chimps are really old, they're too smart) but we managed to get him inside a cat cage to hold him for the anesthesia. We pulled the teeth, and six months later the woman was back.

I didn't really care to go through that fiasco again, and the chimp was now older, smarter and stronger. Charlie liked one of the guys who helped us at the farm. He had a lot of dark hair, and the chimp allowed him to get close and help. The farm hand suggested that we could use a hay drying wagon with holes on the bottom, and come up underneath with a snare to hold Charlie. We took out the chimp's teeth once more, and that was the last we saw of Charlie.

DR. HOPSON SPAYS A MARE

A good client had a beautiful grey mare, about 18 years old, that had been her favorite saddle horse but would chew the fence when it came in heat. She'd have a cycle and go right at the 2x4's until there was nothing left of the whole railing. She was becoming unbearable to be around at these times. The client hated to put the horse to sleep, but didn't know what else to do.

We had a new associate, Dr. Gary Hopson, who came to work for us right out of college. He and I discussed the options of giving hormones or removing the cysts from her ovaries to quiet the horse down. He suggested, "Why don't we do a hysterectomy?" This was unusual, and nobody around here had ever spayed a mare, but we figured we would give it a try. We scheduled it for a Sunday so our office would be closed and we wouldn't be called away on another veterinary case. I gave the anesthesia and our young associate, Dr. Hopson, did the surgery while the mare lay on the owner's lawn. There was a large cyst on her ovary, but I have to say that Gary did a magnificent work of surgery. The mare recovered beautifully, and our client had her, trouble-free, for five more years.

FLUSHED AWAY A FORTUNE

An artificial insemination technician from the next county called and asked if I would look at a 4-H heifer that belonged to a young girl. He had a stack of breeding slips from several failed attempts to get the heifer bred. I told him I couldn't make a special trip that far, but the next time I was out that way doing milk inspections, I would stop in.

I got there and met the nice family who ran the farm; they had nine children at the time, and likely more on the way. Everyone worked together and did their part to help with the chores. The father and mother were at home when I arrived, but the daughter who owned the heifer was at school. The grandmother had helped raise the animal from a calf, and kept pushing the feed to it. The family grew white oats in the middle of the winter to feed the heifer, so she looked more like a beef cow than a registered Holstein. It was easy to see why they couldn't get her bred.

The heifer also had a big cyst on her ovary, which their vet had treated several times, but she still wouldn't conceive. I had asked the artificial breeder if their regular veterinarian had tried a hormone, but he thought the family wouldn't go for that. I knew we needed to do more than remove the cyst to be successful, or they wouldn't like my bill for coming so far out of my territory.

So I said to the father, "See this little bottle? There's another little bottle of water that goes with this dry powder. We're going to have to give it to the heifer if you want to even think about getting her bred." Well, he asked, "Would it work?" I told him, "I can't guarantee it—but it's $72 just for the medicine, and that's not including my charge, so you'd have $150 in this heifer. "My God," he said, "What is that stuff?" I told him, "That's pregnant women's urine." He turned to his wife and said, "Ma, you just pee'd away a fortune!"

My prescription worked, and the heifer did breed. The daughter gave the calf to another 4-H member to continue the program.

COW & STEER IN THE WELL

One morning we were dealt an unusual case: a cow and a steer had fallen into an old well. It was around ten in the morning when I got to the place, and several farmers, local firemen and the extension agent were already assembled, looking over the situation.

The two animals, which looked to be Brown Swiss crosses, had gotten into a well-house by the barn to get out of the bad weather. The gazebo top was still in good shape, but the planks over the well had given way under the weight of the animals. They fell into the opening, which was about 8 feet in diameter, surrounded by walls laid up with stone.

I looked down the well to see that the two animals were displacing the water, taking turns breathing. One would come up and get a breath, and then go down, and the bubbles would come up. Everybody said, "Give 'em a shot." Well, that's what it would have taken to kill them—they both would have died down there. The cow was pregnant and real close to having her calf. The steer was similar in size, and they both had horns. The owner didn't get too excited about the whole event and just did what he needed to do.

The men had already called a tow truck, and cut a hole in the top of the gazebo to put the cable down in. An electrician who was working on the light pole nearby came over to see what was going on. I asked him, "Could we borrow that big wide belt you've got?" He removed all of the tools, and I took the belt with me as some men lowered me into the well. I put the belt around the steer's horns, attached the hook, and the tow truck picked him up out of there. He lay beside the well, just bubbling and gurgling, and looked as if he wasn't going to make it, but I couldn't spend any more time with the steer, since we had to go after the cow. She came out of it well. I put tubes in both animals' stomachs and pumped them out, but the steer was a long time coming around. The fact is, we thought he might have to be butchered. We gave them both penicillin, and the big crowd thought everything turned out pretty good in the end.

The cow had her calf during the night, and was just fine. The steer took a couple of days to recover, but neither animal got pneumonia. I could never get over how the owner of these cattle was so easy-going and completely unconcerned, like it was supposed to happen that way. We really could have lost them both. The owner's wife still talks about that day whenever we see each other.

DEHORNING THE BLACK BULL

About 6:30 one evening, while Shirley was fixing supper and I was playing a little basketball out by the barn, a farmer drove in and said, "I hate to ask you, because I haven't had you to the farm before, but I've got a bull that's gonna die." The farmer had paid a big price for a black Holstein bull and dehorned him that morning. The problem was that the animal would not stop bleeding.

When I got there, I could see that the bull had lost a lot of blood. Back then it was common to leave a stub of the horn showing after dehorning. With cows, baling twine could be tied around the stub, or a rubber band could be twisted around it, and that would stop the bleeding. On bulls over a year old, it doesn't always work since bulls have deeper vessels. A handyman working at the farm had made a plaster cap for the horn to try and stop the bleeding, but it was unsuccessful.

The farmer's teenage son had come out to help. He was cringing while he held the bull's head with the nose leader, and turning away, looking queasy. I asked him now and then, "Is everything all right?" and "Are you OK?" I opened the dehorners real wide, and shifted them around to make a deeper cut. As I pulled out the vessels the bleeding stopped.

After we finished with the one horn, I started to line up the dehorner on the other stub, and the farmer remarked in disbelief, "You're not going to do the other one, are you?" I said, "Sure, you're going to take this bull to the fair, aren't you? Let's match them up."

The bull survived the ordeal and made it to the fair. The farmer became a regular client, and so did his son when he took over the farm. The farmer would talk to me when something important came up. He would never call, he'd just come down to visit; his son was the same way.

SELSUN BLUE DOG SHAMPOO

One of our clients raised Newfoundland dogs, and we used to put selenium sulfide in a bottle for her to give them a bath. It was a terrific cleaner for dog hair, and I purchased this product in bulk through a classmate who worked for Schering Pharmaceuticals. Our client got hooked on it and told me, "I'd like a bigger bottle. It works so good on my dogs I've started using it myself. When I take a shower and wash my hair, it runs down onto the dog, and we both get the benefit." That was before Selsun Blue came on the market—it's pretty much the same thing.

SILO GAS

My daughter Laurie, D.V.M. 1978, and I had been called by a farmer who was one of our regular clients. It was about 1980, in the fall of the year, and he had filled his silo with grass. The farmer had been feeding out of the silo for a few days but stopped, and started to direct-cut grass and feed it to the cows instead. There had been an early fall rain which prevented him from continuing to chop, so he returned to the silo, started the unloader and fed the silage. As the farmer and his father entered the stable after the cows were fed, they saw several cows drop in their stanchions after taking in a mouthful of silage or inhaling the fumes. Some were still conscious but unable to stand.

Laurie and I determined that the cows were poisoned by Nitrogen Dioxide gas which was caused by the worst stages of silage fermentation. To reverse the poisoning we had to get the antidote, Metheline Blue, which was hard to find. Between our supply, the local drugstore and a Ballston veterinarian, we were able to treat the cows by intravenous injection. Several cows died, but we were able to save most of the herd.

Laurie and I were both taught in Large Animal Diagnosis by Dr. Francis Fox at Cornell. On the way home from this call we discussed how Dr. Fox had instructed us to diagnose a case. He would say, "Despite all this book-learning you've had, always remember to use all your senses... stand back and check what you see, smell, hear, taste and touch." This was a good lesson as it made us assess each situation before we got into trouble.

THE FARMER'S WIFE

One of my clients, a dairy farmer who had a small herd, probably stood 5'1" and had married a woman who must've been about 6'2" tall. She was just as skinny as could be, and she liked me because I spent time talking to her. She was always in the barn, and she gave the orders. The couple had an old truck that they used to take their few cans of milk to be pasteurized; they didn't really go that many places. One day when I went the farm to treat a cow the wife wasn't there. I asked the husband, "Where's your wife?" He said, "Oh, you should stop up to the house and see her, she broke her hind leg!"

I guess when you live so close to four-legged animals, you don't think to change the terminology.

24-HOUR TOWING

When one of our associates came to interview, we had a bad prolapse case, and I took him with me on the call. The client ran a sloppy place—cows here, chickens over the top of them, and goats in between. I knew that if our new associate lived through the ordeal, he'd probably stay.

The client who had called would often go down to Albany to get this brewery grain, and come home in his old truck, all tanked up himself, singing at the top of his lungs. He lived on a hill, and if he had to go somewhere, he'd leave his horses down in the hollow with their harnesses on. This way, if anyone had trouble getting up his hill, including the veterinarian, we could just hook the chain on our vehicle and his horses would pull us up—that happened a couple of times. As crazy as we were, we did things like that. The horses knew just what to do—they'd helped get him up that slippery hill a good many times when he came home drunk, singing away.

The man had a standing ad in the local newspaper that he was looking for a Protestant woman to help him on the farm. After a while we asked him why he wanted a Protestant. "Well," he says, "you know these Catholics go to church all day on Sunday, and they don't get nothing done!"

He had an old buck goat that was probably 12 years old. I asked him what he was going to do with this goat. He said, "I'm gonna have you castrate him while you're here, along with a few other jobs." So we did. That winter, while he was fixing a sleigh in the house (with the front bobs and back bobs in pieces), he was boiling up that damn goat! Boy if that wasn't strong—he was gonna have goat meat. We certainly didn't eat anything at his place.

POODLE PUPPY

Two ladies had lost their dog. They came a long way to Burnt Hills to see us when they were clients, and about that same time, an acquaintance of ours had found a poodle puppy in a culvert. The two women rushed up to get that little dog and it just fit the bill. They fussed over it and the puppy filled the void for them, taking the place of their dog that had died. It was a special story with a happy ending. The ladies were so appreciative, that over the years they gave Shirley and me the complete set of James Herriot books.

One of them was inscribed, "To our revered friend, the 'James Herriot of America'—as ever, Alice and Carol."

D.V.M./M.D., SPORTS MEDICINE

One Thanksgiving morning a call came in from a neighbor who said that her dog had caught one of her ducks. She came in right away and the injured duck looked pretty badly hurt. The rib cage was ripped open and the beating heart was fully exposed. A recent Cornell graduate was working with me at this time and we were both on duty. His favorite saying seemed to be "Isn't that terrific," and this is what came out of his mouth when we were examining "Charlie" the duck. Then he asked me, "How are you going to fix this one?" We proceeded to check the internal organs, and clean and suture the wound, all the while thinking it would be a miracle if Charlie survived. In the end, his recovery was uneventful and his owner even showed him at the county fair the next year!

This young veterinarian who had assisted with Charlie the duck had aspirations to go on to medical college. I told him he should pursue it, as I thought he had a great personality for working with people. While he still worked for me, he started going to Union College part-time, eventually finishing up his MD degree and practicing in New York City as an orthopedic surgeon.

A few years later, a friend, who was looking to buy land in the area to build a golf course, was riding along with me on my calls. One of my clients with a small herd of Guernseys was tired of farming and wanted to sell his farm. A deal was made between the men. When the buyer was scouting out the property he had just purchased, he kicked at a woodchuck and ruptured the extensor tendon in his knee. He was in a lot of pain and doctors in the area told him they would not do surgery on it because there might be more involved than the ruptured tendon. One day I casually asked him if he wanted a veterinarian to do it. I told him about my former associate who now was listed on his business card as DVM/MD, Sports Medicine. I called my former associate and he said, "Sure I'd be glad to see your friend, send him down." The surgery was a success with a full recovery for my friend.

When the Olympics were held in Lake Placid in 1980, this orthopedic doctor was on the sports medicine team. Along with three other doctors, he was killed when their plane flew too low coming in to the airport at Lake Placid. It was a tragedy to lose so many gifted people.

TREATING A HUMAN...BLACK SILK STITCHES

In 1962, the last year that our town put snow fences up along the roads, I got my first real experience in treating the human animal. The highway superintendent had hired a new man to help set the posts. One day, when the crew was working on Goode Street in front of the hospital, the superintendent was holding the post and the new man came down with the sledgehammer, splitting his head right open. The superintendent was knocked out cold. Two fellas picked him up under the arms while another one held his feet, and they carried him into our office and set him in a chair.

I had been getting ready for surgery and saw the whole thing happen. I looked the superintendent over as he started to wake up, and all he could mumble was, "Don't cut any hair off." He was more worried about his hair than the bleeding! He had jet-black hair, and I sewed him up with black silk. Somebody said that when he passed away nine years later the sutures were still in there.

NOSEBLEED

We were at our friends' 50th anniversary celebration, when the guest of honor came down with a terrible nosebleed while he was giving a toast. He had a veterinarian on one side of him and a dentist on the other! The dentist and I both tried to help stop the bleeding. I jokingly mentioned that when a horse suffered a nosebleed, we would shove a piece of lemon up its nostril. My bleeding friend said, "Let's give it a try!" We did, and it really worked.

BEAUTY

One of our best mares, Beauty, was close to foaling in early May when a storm came up. Sheets of ice and hail tore the gate down in the partitioned building and Beauty couldn't get back into her stall. She slipped, lost the foal, and couldn't get up, suffering from femeral paralysis. The most she could manage was to raise her front end, and sit up on her haunches. I knew there wasn't much we could do in the way of treatment, and didn't call out to Cornell for advice. I knew what any D.V.M. would have told me: "You know what needs to happen... put her down."

I decided instead that we'd work with her, and we hoisted her back end up with a bucket loader and a couple of tractor belts. This process continued daily for a period of about six weeks. Over that time, her circulation improved, and she got stronger. Eventually she didn't need our assistance to get up, and fully recovered. It was like a miracle to see her get better, and two years later, we bred her back and she had a nice filly.

This incident with Beauty happened toward the end of our 34 years in practice, and was one of our most special cases as I look back. We stuck with it, never gave up, and were blessed with a successful outcome.

THE REST OF THE STORY

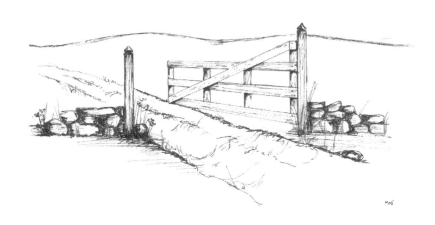

When Shirley and the girls and I had finally settled back in Burnt Hills in 1950 after living in Ithaca, and had established the veterinary practice, we became more involved in the community.

BH-BL ROTARY

As I've said, I was introduced to Rotary while at Cornell, by the Dean, Dr. William Hagan. When I returned from college after my summer internship, the first thing Frank Stevens asked me was, "Is Burnt Hills big enough to have a Rotary club?" "Oh," I said, "sure." While I was away, my father-in-law had shared news of my activities and interests with Al Frieburg, the owner of Burnt Hills Hardware, and in turn, Al, who was on the board of education with Frank Stevens, relayed the news to Frank. Frank and Al had been mulling over the idea, and were excited at the prospect of our chartering a new club together.

We began meeting at our first veterinary hospital, back off the road at the farm, in the fall of 1950 to organize the Burnt Hills-Ballston Lake Rotary Club. There is a plaque on the original building, and a state historical marker at the end of our old lane, which states that the club had its beginnings there.

When we were organizing, there were already three area Rotary clubs, all founded in the 1920's, that were interested in sponsoring our new club. Dr. Harry Hansen and Dr. Post belonged to the Ballston Spa Club, and Percy Dake was District Governor then, from the Saratoga Club, but it was Harley James (along with Joe Martinek and Tony Dorazio), from the Scotia Club who helped us get established. Our 35 charter members were farm-oriented, local business merchants, school professionals and General Electric employees. Our first President, Al Frieburg, received our charter on March 15, 1951.

We are proud of how the Rotary has grown in our community, as well as of our members who live up to the motto of "Service Above Self." There were a record number of new clubs in the capital region in the 1940s and '50s, and ours certainly flourished also.

One of the most significant accomplishments benefiting our town was achieved in cooperation with the Burnt Hills-Ballston Lake Women's Club: founding the Town of Ballston Community Library. The library's first home was in the basement of Our Lady of Grace Church rectory in Ballston Lake. Jessie Townley was head of the Women's Club then, and she and Connie Falconer had discussed the idea of building a Town Library in Burnt Hills. I told Jessie that I thought Rotary would help. She donated the land, and construction began in 1957. The library expanded over the years, and a new one was constructed and opened in 2001. Shirley and I contributed to furnishing the adult lounge at the new library, and were honored with a plaque there in our name.

When I was president of BH-BL Rotary in 1970-71, we started an event that has become a tradition in Burnt Hills: the Apple Pie Festival held each Election Day. The event gets people out to vote, raises funds that go back into our community, and is an opportunity to socialize with friends and neighbors. I thought it would be a good way to celebrate the agricultural area we live in.

Rotary is a wonderful organization and has made a significant impact not just locally, but worldwide. I was proud to be named a Paul Harris Fellow in 1984, and to serve as District Governor in 1986. We were especially pleased when our District raised $15,000 at one event that year for the Polio Plus Campaign, an effort to eradicate this disease around the world.

The Burnt Hills-Ballston Lake Rotary club is made up of many outstanding people, past and present, who have served our community for over 50 years. I was truly humbled when the club established the Stanley "Doc" Garrison Award in 2004 for a life of 'Service Above Self'.

THE CHARLTON SCHOOL

Another organization that has been helping people in our area—for over 100 years—is The Charlton School. It is told that John S. Hawley, a native of Charlton and successful candy manufacturer in New York City, witnessed the poor treatment of two boys caught for stealing while he waited on a train platform. He decided to buy a place where boys could get exercise and work, and founded the Charlton Industrial Farm School for wayward and homeless boys in 1895.

I knew some of the boys there—Sam Benjamin was one of my good friends, Tony Pappas was another one, and so was George Place. I ran cross country with these boys, and we all graduated in 1937. At the time there must've been 35 boys who lived at the Farm School.

They had the most beautiful orchestra over there and performed on Saturday nights—all the boys learned to play an instrument. From our house it was just one mile cross-lots. All the boys, even the little ones, had suits and went to church in Charlton. The bigger boys took care of them.

There was a horrible fire at the Farm School in 1938 and all the buildings were destroyed. Funding for the school went into escrow, and the courts decided there was more need for a facility for girls than boys. When it was rebuilt, it opened in 1955 as a residential treatment center and school for troubled teenage girls. At the time of the fire the boys were dispersed to other homes and residential facilities.

The campus of the school occupies only fifty acres of the three hundred-acre property. I rented and cropped the farmland, and was a trustee on the board for over 50 years, serving as president from 1971-74.

During that time, a nephew of the founder, John Hawley, contacted the school. He ran a coffee plantation in Guatemala and was looking to buy some dairy cattle. He understood that there was a veterinarian on the board, and wanted me to recommend a breed that could withstand the hot climate. Another board member, Harold Magnussen, sold him some Brown Swiss heifers, and we were invited, along with our wives, to visit this unique country in Central America. It was quite a trip and our experiences could fill a chapter of their own!

The rural setting of the Charlton School brings the world of nature and the outdoors into the lives of the students. Shirley and I were pleased to help fund the building of an Adirondack lean-to which is near the school's pond, nature trails, wildlife feeding stations, and the Alplaus creek.

THE NEW
BURNT HILLS VETERINARY HOSPITAL

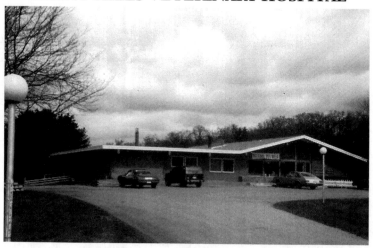

1961

After 11 years of practicing veterinary medicine at the barn location, Shirley and I built a new hospital, at the front of our property on Goode Street, in 1961. The balance between large and small animal care had now reversed—our practice was 30% large animal, and 70% small animal.

When we built the new hospital we were aware of what needed to be done differently from the old one, and made 10 inside exercise runs with insulated glass and drains. A climate-controlled room allowed us to work efficiently without getting out in the cold.

We used our small clinical refrigerator to keep vaccines and other things cool. It became a practical joke, especially when new vet students came for the summer, to take a drink from a batch of iced tea that was sitting beside beakers of urine samples.

OUR FARM

When we moved the hospital from the barn to the front of the property, we made an apartment out of the old hospital, and several young couples used our farm to get their start in the dairy business. Wayne and Janice Arnold were the first to farm there, followed by our daughter Linda and her husband Jay Walter. Tom and Debbie Johnson were the next couple to follow suit—Debbie also had a two-year vet tech degree and worked for us at the hospital. These families all stayed for two or three years before going on to farms of their own. Shirley and I continued to raise hay and grain, some dairy heifers, and Belgian draft horses.

Over the years, we have seen many changes on our 160-acre farm, and within the community. In the late 40's early 50's we sold the orchard and horse pasture to Kenneth Sack, who built Orchard Terrace and Woodside Drive with many fine homes on the property. This sale, along with the crops from the rest of our land, helped finance my education. In the 1960's we were approached by the school district to sell 28 acres bordering Scotchbush and Jenkins Roads. We agreed, and it is still open land.

Thirty years later, Westview Manor was created on our property, a 25-lot development surrounding Goodman

Court, Katherine Drive, and an extension of Woodside Drive. Next, we built an 11-lot development on David's Lane and Miller Court, on the east side of Goode Street. The remaining 17 wooded acres off of David's Lane was divided into three large lots.

We're proud of the way the land has developed into a beautiful neighborhood of nice family homes and we credit John Gay for his expertise in laying out the property. In June of 2000, our granddaughter Darlene purchased our farmhouse, and later, in 2004, she bought the original big barn which had been renovated into a large single apartment.

GROWTH

While our land developed, so did our entire area. The population of our town has increased four-fold in my lifetime. I was pleased to chair the ceremonies to dedicate the "new" post office in 1961, which was outgrown in 40 years, and has been replaced now with a much larger building further north on Route 50. I was also honored to have a part in renaming the former Burnt Hills-Ballston Lake Central School building in 1967, as Francis L. Stevens Elementary—recognizing my mentor and friend.

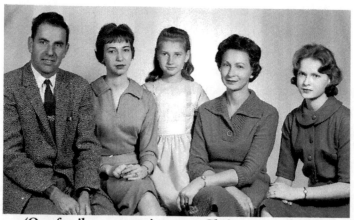

(Our family was growing too—Christmas card 1960)

MORE FARMS!

Along with our home farm, we had the opportunity to work land on other farms in the area, and ended up buying four of them over the years. It turned out all right, but was probably Shirley's biggest nightmare at the time since she kept track of all the bookwork.

We leased the farm at the Charlton School on Lakehill Road, and in 1955, the Ward sisters proposed selling 55 acres of their land just down the road from the school. We kept the barn, and they kept the house. Ten years later, Lauren Rowledge wanted to know if I'd like to buy his farm of 64 acres that joined the school's acreage.

LaRue Creek bordered this block of property on one side, and the Alplaus Creek on other side. We could move cows from Rowledge's to the Charlton School through the culvert underneath the road, and did that many times while the kids who helped us on the farm rode their horses to herd the cattle.

The Miller farm (no relation to Shirley's family), on Devil's Lane, didn't have the best buildings, but the two silos there were choice. Two years went by, and the sign was still up to sell 176 acres when we decided to buy it.

We also worked the Cappiello farm on Route 50 when Tom Johnson and Tom Miller were working for me.

The last farm we bought, and sold soon after, was one on Farm-to-Market Road in the town of Halfmoon. This was originally owned by Joshua Anthony, and still has the name J.H. Anthony on the barn's slate roof. Joshua's cousin, Susan B. Anthony, spent summers at the farm, which also operated a spice mill at that time.

DRAFT HORSES

Since I had been brought up with draft horses, I wanted to get a pair of "farm chunks" as they called them back in my father's day. I talked with Dr. Francis Fox, my professor at Cornell, who had spent a year at Ohio State Veterinary College. He advised me to talk to the Dean at Ohio State who was familiar with the spring sales at the fairgrounds in Columbus.

These sales were usually held in early February, and attended by many horsemen including Amish farmers who brought their animals in for auction. I did go, and found on that first visit some 800 draft horses consigned.

It was some time into the sale before I found a team that suited me in price, conformation, and disposition, and I thought were worth bidding on. A pair of matched blonde Belgian mares, Molly and Joan, came in the ring; I remember they were the 19th team to be sold that day, and I bid enough to bring them home. The Amish man who owned this team, Mose Yoder, offered to sell me their collars and harnesses too. Just like that we were in the draft horse business!

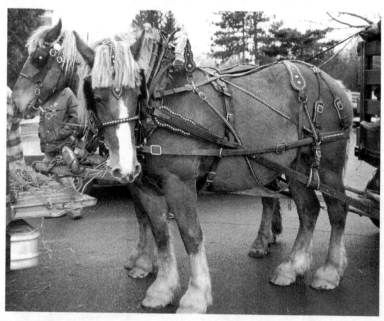

Our first team of Belgians from Ohio, Molly and Joan

We became friends with the Yoders and sent the mares back to their farm in Ohio to be bred each year. Mose had a sound stallion that provided extra income from breeding. These mares each foaled four years in succession giving us eight beautiful offspring. When the mares were bred back after the fourth foaling, Mose wrote me a letter saying that he wanted to buy them back.

We were able to visit another Amish horseman from Ohio over the years, and got a first-hand glimpse of Amish life. Johnny Miller was a very clever farmer who built and raised his own barns with his neighbors. His farm was really impressive: neat and clean and taken care of. His wife, Mary, was a little short woman who was always pregnant as long as we knew her. Johnny and Mary had 10 kids: twins in the first pregnancy, then six girls in row, followed by two boys. Mary was 32 years old then. The women milked the cows and the men did the fieldwork with horses. They had a beautiful garden right next to the house, and the little kids did all the gardening work. Children went to the one-room schools when they were seven years old, and stayed through the eighth grade; formal schooling for the Amish is only a part of the learning necessary to prepare for the adult world. Any girl who was big enough could run a sewing machine.

The Amish usually keep to themselves, but are very friendly if they get to know you and like you. Shirley and I stayed at the Millers' house one night, and they killed the biggest rooster they had and got a chunk of ice to make homemade ice cream.

Johnny was short and lean. I can still see him hoist that heavy harness and throw it on the horse, which didn't dare move. His horses were all well-trained from daily work.

The Amish don't drive, but once somebody brought the Millers in a van to our place in Burnt Hills to look at our horses. They liked the nice feet our horses had. They didn't shoe their horses, and the shale in their area is tough on the horses' feet.

BUYING AN 8-HORSE HITCH WAGON

Another time, I went to the Columbus sale with my son-in-law Jay, to purchase a hitch wagon for our matched team of Belgians. There was one advertised in a flier we received that would be the showcase of the sale. It was a beautiful piece of work, with smaller front wheels, and larger rear wheels with three poles for four teams of horses. The front team or lead team does not need a pole between them—they're the smartest team on the hitch. The paint job was several coats of green lacquer finished to perfection. Rumor had it that the owner had spent three winters getting this wagon assembled like the original old fashion types. The bidding started and Jay and I stood in a used horse-drawn manure spreader to keep a better view. I bid as the starter, followed by a couple more, and soon the auctioneer struck it off to us.

This show wagon went from county fairs, to state fairs, to the veterinary convention, Albany's tri-centennial celebration parade, and the Ellis Hospital parade. It was also in the Travers Parade in Saratoga celebrating the Centennial of the NYS Veterinary Medical Society (1990). The Travers Committee was originally established to celebrate the Travers race, and to raise funds for equine research programs at the New York State College of Veterinary Medicine at Cornell.

DRAFT HORSE CLUB

In the 1970's, my fellow Draft Horse enthusiasts and I decided to start a club, so Stanley Rickard, Bob Anderson, Herb Peters, Wendell Saunders and I chartered the Eastern Regional Draft Horse Association. I took a term serving as president, and Shirley and I hosted the annual club picnic for several years.

We've probably had 50 Belgians over a period of 20 years, and many stories involving draft horses and their teamsters stay in my memory. One in particular was an occasion at the Cobleskill Fair. Bob Anderson, who trained many of my horses, and I were given the opportunity to drive Herb Peters' four-horse hitch. If you have seen Herb sit on that seat with four or six-up, and no words pass from his lips, you know how we felt trying to make them maneuver on the track during the driving contest. Stanley Rickard, who was judging the class, was so upset at how we attempted to handle the challenge, that he was going to have us ushered off the track; you do not drive Herb Peters' horses with words, just grunts. If you asked any of these men to help you harness, drive or aid you in any type of work, they were more than willing.

I have treated many cases of injuries and colics for these horsemen friends and have a good idea how much their animals mean to them. I remember treating a mare for Herb Peters that was close to foaling and had colic. She was down in the box stall at one of those ungodly hours that mares have colic, with a temperature of 103 degrees, yellow mucous membranes, and thrashing for her life. Working at the front of the horse first, I put a stomach tube down through her nose and gave some Epsom salts, then went to the back end with some ivory soap to get things moving. Perhaps what the last veterinarian did for the horse was finally starting to kick in, because after about two hours, she was on her feet and had delivered a live foal.

I got back at Herb for making me work at that awful hour by calling him early one morning at the end of March, and asking him if he wanted to plant oats. He thought I was off my beam, saying he had eight inches of snow at his place! He came down, brought a four-horse evener, and we planted three acres of oats with two teams of horses. One team was Bernie Palmer's and the other was mine. Chet Orzolek came behind with his pair and cultipacked the ground which improves the soil-to-seed contact. Months later, we threshed the oats with an old fashioned thresher one Sunday at Chet's, and drew a crowd of both young and old spectators.

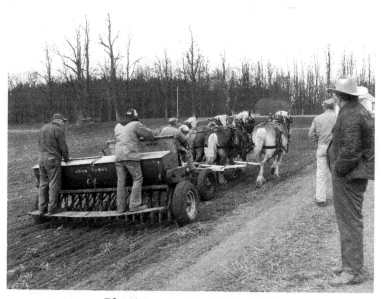

Planting oats March 27, 1981
at the Rowledge Farm, Sweetman Road, Charlton
Herb Peters driving the two teams, Bernie Palmer (left) checking the grain drill, Bill Muraskas riding (at right), Ed Button supervising (back, right) and yours truly (front, right).

The club held annual Plow Days and Silo Fills at various farms and participated in the Ice Harvest at Miller's Mills each year. Members pulled floats in parades, and showed animals at all the fairs around. We had a lot of fun in our draft horse days, going to the sales in Cortland, as well as trips to Ohio, Pennsylvania and Indiana.

In 1980 our town historian, Kathy Briaddy, asked us to help with a 200th Anniversary reenactment of the British-Indian Invasion. We brought the horses to the Firemen's Grove for the Town of Ballston's Heritage weekend.

RETIREMENT?

The veterinary practice had been the biggest part of our lives for 34 years. Selling it was not an easy moment to face, but when we made the transition in January 1984, the responsibilities to the clients, employees, and running of the hospital were no longer ours. Shirley and I adjusted pretty well to retirement, but there were many times we missed our routine of so many years, and most of all, the contact with our clients.

Upon my retirement, I was honored to receive the Veterinarian of the Year Award for 1984 from the Capital District Veterinary Medical Society. This recognition for "dedicated service to my community and profession" was a highlight of my career, in addition to serving as President of the New York State Veterinary Medical Society in 1970-71.

The year I ran for president of the State Society, a classmate of mine, Dr. Stanley Aldrich, from Babylon N.Y., was also a nominee. We were good friends and together decided that regardless of who won, we were in agreement that the State Society must be moved from Utica to Albany. As it turned out, I was elected in 1971 and Dr. Aldrich won in 1972. We both worked to establish the office in Albany where it is close to the state governing process. Dr. Aldrich went on to become president of the American Veterinary Medical Association in 1980-81, and did a great job to promote veterinary medicine.

In 1984 I also enjoyed a wonderful retirement party at the Lower Mohawk Club, organized by my colleague, Frank Rapp, D.V.M. Many associates attended whom I hadn't seen in years!

Looking back, Shirley and I agree that selling the practice was the best decision we could have made. It gave me the time to pursue farming and work with the horses, and we also had time for ourselves to travel, visiting Europe, Central America, Canada, and many places in the U.S. including Alaska. Most of all, it allowed us time to enjoy the closeness of family and friends. We learned that we must always make changes in our lives work for us, and not let them become a crisis.

Retirement is a state of mind, and ours has been busy-keeping us feeling young. Shirley graduated from Fulton Montgomery Community College in 1987, with a degree in Visual Fine Arts. It was a great experience for her being a college student in her sixties. For the past 10 years, Shirley has enjoyed being close to nature in our cabin in the woods by a stream, and I have bounced back and forth from there to Burnt Hills, slowing down, but only once in a while.

On March 15, 1998, our family and friends came together to celebrate my 80th birthday at the Elks Club in Ballston Lake, which was a special day I will always remember.

In 2000 we celebrated the town of Ballston's agricultural heritage and the centennial anniversary of our barn in Burnt Hills, with a barbecue and tours of the restored barn. A historic marker was unveiled, and guest speakers at the dedication ceremony included Nathan Rudgers, NYS Commissioner of Agriculture and resident of Burnt Hills, along with Robert VanVorst, grandson of the original owner of the farm, Charles VanVorst.

The women of the Burnt Hills United Methodist Church were our guests that day, as they had provided dinner each week for nearly 50 years to the Burnt Hills-Ballston Lake Rotary Club. The women from this same church in 1900 were also remembered, as they put on a meal for the men as they raised the barn on Goode Street 100 years before.

We celebrated my 50th Reunion at the Cornell Veterinary College in 2000, and the Burnt Hills-Ballston Lake Rotary Club's 50th the following year.

One of the best celebrations of all, was my 87th birthday dinner this spring (2005), with family all around the table at my granddaughter's, the farmhouse on Goode Street in Burnt Hills, where I was born.

Our Family

Our three daughters each have two grown children, so we are blessed with six grandchildren and two great-grandchildren. Youngest daughter, Laurie worked with me for eight years, and lives in California with her husband Brian Harms, where she plans to practice veterinary medicine. They have two sons, Matthew and Derek. Our middle daughter Linda and her husband Jay Walter live in Sauquoit, NY. They have a daughter Amy, and a son, Mike. Our oldest daughter, Diane, and her husband Bob Condit live at Friends Lake, NY. Her children Darlene and Garry each have one son; Evan and Dewitt. Our great grandson, Evan Bickford is the sixth generation to live on the home farm.

REFLECTIONS

Looking back over my 87 years, there were many gates, opening and closing, that led to a full and satisfying life. Some were difficult to struggle through, and many seemed like fate forcing the decisions, but there were always opportunities and people urging me on to better things.

Although we can't possibly mention all of the wonderful people who had a part in the success of the Burnt Hills Veterinary Hospital and shared our lives, we feel we need to give special thanks to:

Judy Brenner, Jean Carr, Frances Heath, Rachel Hubbell, Pat Pustolka, Kathy Jette Sisler, Jean Stansfield and Ann Yager–Office Staff, Debbie Healy Johnson and Lyn Mackerer Clatworthy –Veterinary Technicians, Drs. Joseph Bryan, Donald Fox, Gary Hopson, Frank Martoranna, and Sondra Wand–Veterinarians,

Our three girls–Diane, Linda and Laurel,
Our grandchildren and great-grandchildren,
Stan's brother and sisters, and
Shirley's brother and family

During the 1950's and 60's, when our kids were growing up on Goode Street, we had a community of family and close friends all around us. Most of the children were cousins as my two sisters and Shirley's brother had built homes on part of our farm. Even Shirley's parents lived next door to us and were Gram and Gramps to all. Jean Stansfield, and her daughter Hilarie and son John, were close friends and Jean came to work for us in the hospital when her husband Leonard died. Shirley and Jean were like sisters over the years, helping each other in times of need.

The home farm on Goode Street has always been the center of my world. It provided a solid foundation for my childhood with my family, and then for Shirley and I to raise our children. It also gave us the opportunity to pursue the practice of veterinary medicine and farming, which directly involved us in our wonderful community of friends in and around Burnt Hills, Saratoga County, New York.

When our family and friends came together in 1998 to celebrate my 80th birthday, they put together an album of photos and memories, which I treasure. The following letters are just a few from the album:

March 1998

To Stan and all his Family,

First of all, I'm extremely sorry that I have to miss such an important occasion for such a remarkable man. Punky and I are still in the sunny West Texas area and won't return to the Northeast until April. Regardless of the weather, I'm sure March 15th will be a sunny day in Ballston Lake.

I first met Stan in early July 1960, the Fourth to be exact, on a very hot day. I was inquiring about an ad for employment. After a very auspicious call we took together for a bovine prolapse, we had some of Shirley's wonderful cooking, and within two weeks I was working full time for, I think, eighty dollars a week. What I learned in two years about veterinary medicine, and farming, and bulldozer operation, and human nature in general was unbelievable. I couldn't have had a better job or a better home.

I lived in the basement of Stan and Shirley's house and ate my meals with Shirley's Mom and Dad. I think I had the best of both worlds except, maybe, for the one morning when I woke up and stepped into three or four inches of water! I was always treated like one of the family, that is for sure. In fact, I still feel that I'm, in some way, a part of the Garrison family.

I'm not going to tell any "stories" about Stan. First of all it would take up too much space. But I do remember many events and just some things that tell a bit about this giant of a man.

I remember when Dr. Frank Rapp had an auto accident and was out of commission for awhile. Stan said one of us should go down and help him out for a bit, so I went every day for almost a week (I think) and did treatments, took office calls, etc., with Frank's staff. I'm not sure that would happen today.

I remember Stan building his own swimming pool- concrete walls and all, from scratch. Naturally he did the dozer work!

I remember that Stan seemed to make more animals well with less medicine than anyone I've ever met before or since.

We worked at the time with general office hours and no appointments. Clients would wait for hours and never get upset or leave, as long as they could eventually get to see their shining knight. Stan had such rapport with clients—just wonderful—such faith! For two years I observed, studied and analyzed Dr. Stan and his ways and handling of clients. I finally decided that there was just no way of duplicating his bedside manner, because there is only one Dr. Stan Garrison.

I feel most fortunate and really blessed to have worked with Stan, to have lived with his family, and to have known and loved the Stan Garrison you are honoring on March 15th.

Most Sincerely,

Donald C. Fox

March 15, 1998

Stan,

We have shared a lot of experiences in 36 years as fellow Rotarians. My first Rotary assignment was to judge a pet show at the Library with the assurance that "All you have to do is pass out ribbons, Stan Garrison will handle the animals." Nobody warned me that you would probably be a half hour late! In a mob of complaining kids, barking dogs and squalling cats you finally came to my *rescue. I was trying to determine the "cat with the longest tail" award by using a 12-inch ruler on some very unhappy and uncooperative cats!*

We also shared the misery of trying to solve the problems created by our Argentine exchange student, Graciela. Her boyfriend's angry father came to my office to "wring my neck" first, after which he planned to do yours. I suggested he take you first, since you were the club president and I didn't wish to usurp your privileges.

Stan, I have a lot of good memories of our association, Rotary conferences, the first Apple Pie Festival, your great year as District Governor when we raised $15,000 for Polio Plus, and my Paul Harris award which was largely your doing, I'm sure.

Your 80th birthday is a milestone in the full and very productive life of a respected and highly regarded member of the community in which you were born. You have been a great contributor and with your present energy and vigor, I'm sure there is more to come!

Thanks and best wishes,

Bill Sewell

Each of our daughters shared their special memories in letters for my 80th birthday album:

Dear Dad,

Do you remember when you tore the roof off the old farmhouse in Ithaca and we all prayed it wouldn't rain until you got a new one on? I always imaged that the upstairs tenants spent those nights staring up at the open sky.

Do you remember finding horseradish growing in the backyard by the barn in Ithaca? Seems that I remember Mom trying to grind it up for sauce and that it was some strong stuff! We probably could have bottled it and made a fortune.

I remember getting locked in the hen house with Carol Hammond and I thought I'd probably spend the rest of my life there. I was so scared! Carol's brother, Arty, thought it was very funny.

I know you remember eating eggs four or five times a week because Katherine gave Mom all her cracks. You know, it's a wonder any of us still like eggs.

Scoop Lewis is a wonderful memory too. I remember him living with us at the farmhouse, and then at the apartment. He carried me out of the building the morning of the fire, remember?

Oh God, do you remember my friend Priscilla? She had a parrot and a little brother. Her mother tied her brother out to a tree in their back yard when she didn't want to have him under foot. I recall playing "step on a crack, break your mother's back" with her. We had the worst old broken sidewalks and steps and old iron handrails around the block on Stewart Avenue.

And that poor, sad hound dog that I decided must be homeless. Linda and I walked all the way to the Veterinary College to find you. I remember Lindy losing her shoe right in the middle of the rotary and having to stop to help her put it back on. It's a wonder Mom hadn't filed a missing children's report on that one. Also, how about when I went to visit a friend and boarded the wrong bus to come home and got lost. Or the time I ran away from home with Carol Hammond and you all had to come and find us.

How about the time when I was very small that I decided to take a walk down the farm lane and go visit Aunt Mabel. She was painting the sash of her kitchen window from a step ladder and drinking iced tea.

The trips we took back and forth from Burnt Hills to Ithaca—they were long for a little kid, but I remember having a wonderful time singing songs and listening to you whistle. Every time I hear "I Want to Dance with the Dolly with a Hole in her Stocking," I think of bouncing along in one old car or truck or another. Nobody could whistle as good as my father!

I remember having you drop me off at nursery school at Cornell and kindergarten in Ithaca. I remember my first grade teacher—her breath smelled like cream of mushroom soup! I think that was when I got the health report that said my chest was slightly concave and I was pigeon-toed. I was skinny and shy, but she scared me so bad, I wet my pants one day, and Mom had to come to my rescue.

I remember when you got kicked and broke your leg. I couldn't figure our why you were going to live at the fraternity house instead of staying with us. That was the same day that Mom was fretting about not having any money and I thought I had all the answers. I told her, "Well, why don't you just write a check?"

You graduated in 1950 and I was not quite seven years old, so all of the above memories are clouded by a child's mind and almost fifty years. I know that the best times and memories are not necessarily from the good years, but from the years we spent getting to the good years. We made such wonderful history back then and I'm so glad we can all still look back on those days and remember the fun and friends that went along with all the hardships.

In case you're wondering, I think you're still the best whistler!

Love, Diane

Happy Birthday Dad,

What a joy it has been for our family to have this 80th Birthday Party for you. We have all come to appreciate you much more as the unique and exciting person that you are, and we have savored the varied aspects of your life. We all marvel at how your energy and adventures have enriched our lives and stretched us as individuals, as we have traveled the road of life together as a family. I would like to share some of my special memories of childhood for your scrapbook.

Thanks for Peppy, our St. Bernard, while you were in college. I remember that there were 14 puppies in the litter and that because you saved the mother dog, they gave you a puppy. Diane and I had stayed with Norma and Alan the night before you brought her home and we all ran over to see her the next morning as fast as we could. A favorite family story happened when Peppy grew too big to sleep behind the bathtub and you had to take the bathtub out to get her out.

Diane, Laurie and I had the best time with our Welsh Mountain pony, Frisco, which you bought for us on Sunnyside Avenue in Scotia. For hours, all the kids in the neighborhood would practice running up and jumping on his back or side, just like all the cowboy movies we saw. He was so patient and good to us. When he finally died, you buried him in the woods for us, with a huge boulder as his grave marker.

I still remember selling raccoon skins to some man who lived in a little shack by the railroad track. You took care of some unusual creatures as a veterinarian when I was tagging along. The lion with the traveling circus, and chimpanzee who needed his teeth worked on. Who could record the number of calls that I went on with you. You always had little jobs for me to do, so I would learn and feel important. When I became a teenager, you'd let me drive and always gave me advice like, "lock your doors if you stop at a railroad track" and "don't pass a truck going up a hill, it could overrun you on the way down." The family would often accompany you on a call and we would stop for dinner; I think I would always have a shrimp cocktail.

Remember the Confederate money I put in the scrapbook? That happened on a Thanksgiving Day when many extended family members took a long walk. We found this money in an abandoned place way off the beaten path. We all had a wonderful time, and we were sure that we had stumbled onto hidden treasure.

At 10 years of age, with your encouragement and assistance, I accumulated my own little herd of calves. We bought my Jersey from Wesley Martin, the Guernsey from John Lane, my favorite, my Brown Swiss who I named Linda, from Lou Weston, the Ayrshire who I bid on and bought myself at John Belott's auction for $35.00 (while waiting for you), and of course my Holstein calf. It was always exciting bringing them home in the front seat of the car by my feet, in a burlap bag. When I was 12 and Jay was 13 we had our cows next to each other at the county fair. My experience raising calves certainly proved very useful to us for the twenty years that we ran our dairy farm.

Of course the most notorious event you involved me in was with Babe and the Freihofer delivery wagon. I am so very proud of you for all you have accomplished—especially recently with repairing and beautifying the Sweetman Cemetery. You have made a lot of things happen for the betterment of Burnt Hills that I know wouldn't have happened otherwise.

Thanks, Dad for being such a faithful father. I have always been able to count on your love and support. Thanks for everything! I'm looking forward to many more years of great adventure with the best Dad a girl could ever have.

Love always,
Lindy

Dear Dad,

I wanted to relay some memorable events in my life for your 80th birthday album.

The earliest one is of having a stomach "bug" and sitting curled up on your lap on the naughahyde lounger. We were by the book-shelf and fireplace. That was a great chair, cool and smooth—and always had coins that had fallen down inside from your pockets! We weren't doing much, but you were just taking time to be with me.

I was a little older when I found myself riding a new pony down the road with you hanging on to her through the car window as you drove down the road to home. That was "Cindy," I think, and she delivered a nice spotted foal one morning before school in the old calf barn. Can you imagine someone bringing a pony home on today's roads like this?

At about this age I had a great present—the longest tree swing a girl could have. Between those two grand oaks, and from side to side, wrapping that rope around the trees, I could dream for hours. Sometimes you'd rush in for lunch from a large animal call, wash up, and be off to office hours. And I could just swing in the sun!

Another incident that sticks in my memory, although not spec-tacular is special. On our train trip to California in 1962 you and I got off in Salt Lake City to find a "hole in the wall" diner and we had some kind of salty chicken soup. We had no idea where we were (probably not the best part of town) and we just made it back to the train on time!

Of course my best present was my pony Cherokee. For 20 years he was a part of my life. Through him I experienced freedom and being outdoors in the woods and on the trails.

My story wouldn't be complete without thanking you for inspiring me to become a veterinarian. You and Dr. Poppensick were instru-mental in helping me get accepted to Cornell Veterinary College.

Thanks for all of these and many more great memories.

Love,
Laurie

Winding Down

Written by Stewart Rockwell, D.V.M.,
a classmate from Veterinary College in 1950
who was also a District Governor of Rotary.
He and his wife, Mary, live in Emmaus, PA.

Veterinary medicine has been my life.
It's involved the whole family, children and wife.
They worked in the office and went on calls,
Had to put up with smelly coveralls.
A foaling mare or a downer cow,
Can't wait 'til later, it had to be now.
Early in the morning or late at night,
And then some times by lantern light.
Weather may be cold or could be hot,
They have to be treated, weather or not.
Of the many animals, large or small,
Over the years I've done it all.
Perhaps not an elephant or kangaroo,
With those I wouldn't know what to do.
I've gotten older and the time has come
When doing those things is no longer fun.
I've enjoyed practice and made many friends,
That part of my life has come to an end.
I like to garden and see things grow,
There are lots of places I intend to go.
I'm looking forward to the next few years,
When once again I'll probably shift gears.

A LIVING LEGACY

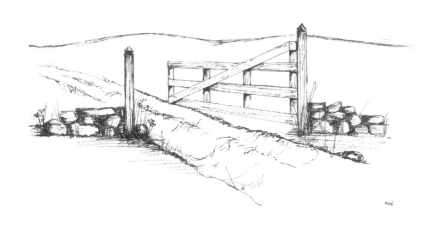

"Doc" Garrison and the
Burnt Hills Veterinary Hospital
–A Living Legacy

by Pete Farrell, D.V.M., Burnt Hills, N.Y.

As senior veterinary students at Cornell's Veterinary College in February of 1982, Mike Rach and I were actively seeking employment for after graduation in June. The annual Cornell Conference for Veterinarians was the best place to look, because it was when all the hospital owners who needed to recruit new doctors would be in town to interview prospects. It was an uncomfortable time for some of us, because we were competing with our friends and classmates for the best available positions.

My own search was very focused. The Burnt Hills Veterinary Hospital seemed like just the right spot for me. I wanted to work in a practice that cared for both farm animals as well as pets. I wanted it to be a progressive, interesting place to work. And I wanted there to be several doctors on staff to share ideas, thoughts and responsibilities. After having a talk with Doc, I was even more certain that Burnt Hills was the place for me. There were four of us that were very interested in working for Doc, but he was only looking for one. After speaking with all of us, he decided he would actually hire two of us. So we individually made the trek up from Ithaca to visit the Hospital and see what it was really like.

Doc was in constant motion. He would do a spay, then see a sick dog, then mow a field of hay, then check on his pregnant Belgian mare, then make a farm call to check a cow that wasn't eating. His schedule was somewhat chaotic, because he tried to take care of his own farms and horses, do his farm calls, and be in the hospital. The only way his staff could keep track of him was with the two-way radio. If there was a client with a dog that was waiting for him and he had to leave to go to a farm, he'd invite them to ride along. I knew right from the start that it would be hard to keep up with Doc.

Mike and I were each offered a position at the hospital in April, so we came up to visit Doc again. He showed us around Burnt Hills, introduced us to staff and local farmers, and showed us places we could live. We were sold. We both joined on and were set to start in late June of 1982.

It was a whirlwind. Both Mike and I struggled to learn as much as we could from Doc and his daughter Laurie, who had graduated from Cornell in 1978. Doc used to say, "You won't find that on page 99," referring to some bit of crucial information that he had just imparted. Our educational experience had been that the "Cornell Way" was the only right way. We quickly learned that there were other very effective ways of getting things done. We garnered Doc's manner with clients as well. He would tell people straight up, what was wrong and what needed to be done. But he empathized and would hug folks when they lost their loved one, and many times would try to find them a new pet right then and there. His hands-on compassionate way with clients clearly engendered much trust from them.

About a year after we started working for Doc, he approached me and Mike with the news that he was ready to sell the hospital and that he would like to sell it to us. We were stunned. We hadn't gotten comfortable with doing veterinary medicine and surgery yet, and now he wanted us to take over running the hospital! We were scared and lacked any knowledge of how to purchase the hospital, much less run it well after purchasing it. So we dragged our heels. We didn't get serious about his request until he made it clear that if we weren't going to purchase the hospital, he would go looking for someone else. After the first prospective buyer was given his tour of the hospital, we got busy.

By January of 1984, Mike and I were the new owners of the Burnt Hills Veterinary Hospital. As a parting gift to us, Doc had purchased a brand new farm vet truck for us and presented it at the annual Christmas Party. He wanted to give us every opportunity to succeed.

Much has changed in the ensuing years. Many of the dairy farmers Doc had taken care of took advantage of the dairy buy-out *program. In 1985, we stopped doing farm calls because our area was changing from a farming community to a suburban community. We began to offer more evening hours, and increased Saturday hours to make the hospital available to families with two working parents. As we grew, we hired new associates, and staff. When we started, Mike and I were the only full time doctors with Laurie working part time. We had a staff of seven. We now have seven full time doctors, three part time doctors, and a support staff of 60.*

Doc had been told that building his hospital in his hometown was a very bad idea. He was also told that building the modern facility he did in 1961 was foolish and that he would never be able to pay for it. Thankfully, he didn't listen. Doc started with the idea that taking good care of people's animals, whether they were farm animals or pets, was something they wanted. He was right. Our clients' expectations for care of their pets are that they want the same level of care they expect for themselves. This requires that we constantly reinvent ourselves, learning and providing new services, purchasing the latest equipment, going to continuing education meetings, reevaluating current procedures. This was the philosophy Doc imbued us with. It was his approach and became our own. The success we have enjoyed is in large measure due to the influence that Doc had on two young new graduate veterinarians back in 1982.

Who knows what the future of the hospital will be? Will we have to continue to expand our facility? Will we purchase CT scanners or MRI machines? Will we hire specialists? The foundations upon which we are building, and received from Stan Garrison, continue to guide our future endeavors. The Burnt Hills Veterinary Hospital will continue as a legacy to Stan and Shirley Garrison and provide "the best of care for the best of friends" to any and all.

Part of Doc's legacy was his inspiration to young people over the years to follow their dreams. Dr. Trish Herr's introduction to this story is a touching tribute and testimony to Doc's positive influence as is the following shared by Shirley:

Many young boys came to work for Stan on the farm over the years. It was always a special pleasure for him to help them pursue their ambitions toward their career goals. One young man in particular, Frank Martoranna, needed farm experience in order to apply to veterinary college. Frank worked two summers for Stan, mostly on the farm, but also rode with him on large animal calls. Stan was pleased to write a letter of recommendation for Frank when he applied to Cornell, and was very proud of him when he graduated with his D.V.M. Frank was thankful for the encouragement Stan had given him and for all of his learning experiences from Burnt Hills.

The excerpt below is from a letter written by a local young woman who followed a similar path to a successful medical career. When she was a teenager her mother, Sally, commented to Doc, "You've not only been a role model to boys, but also to my daughter."

You were a fundamental part of my early years. I remember running to the barn to help clean the stalls and braid the horses' tails for the Charlton parade. You always put a smile on my face showing me where to stand to avoid a swift kick, along with all the other essential "how-to's". I remember you calling Dad when a new foal was about to arrive so that I could come to watch. It was such a miracle! I also remember our little dog being sick and you operating on her while I got to watch. I should have been sad, but it was so cool watching you work and having you share with me what you were doing, that I wasn't. (I did hope that you would remember to put all her parts back in when you were done) I'm happy to say she had another 15 good years after that day. I could go on forever, but I think I'll end here. Thank you for all the wonderful memories!
With love, Kristin Gay

From the author...

About a year ago Doc was telling me that he had given up on the idea of writing his book. "The project is too big for Shirley and me, and we're too close to it. Maybe it's not of interest to the younger generations." He had shared some of his memories at the "Farm Life Stories Gatherings," which a friend and I were holding in several towns throughout our county, and I knew these stories were too precious to just fall by the wayside. I encouraged him to pursue the book, and offered to help; it wasn't long before I was writing it.

This book is special to me for several reasons—not only am I interested in preserving our local agricultural history, but some of Doc's stories speak to my own heritage. I am proud to say we're related: my maternal grandfather, Earl Garrison, and Stan were cousins. Coincidentally, my paternal great-grandfather, Stephen H. Merchant, was a neighbor of Stan's and had a profound influence on his life.

Several of my relatives appear in these stories before I was even born. My grandfather, David Palmer, drove the "rural school bus"—Merchant's farm delivery truck, when the potato rolled out at Stan's feet as it stopped to pick him up. He is the same farmer who called on Stan to save his bull from bleeding to death, and my father, Bernie Palmer, was the teenage son who assisted.

I grew up on my family's dairy farm in the town of Ballston, and can remember Doc "whisking in" countless times over the years. He would do the routine blood work and give shots prior to the county fair each summer, as well as perform a harrowing operation to sew up a cow's ruptured milk vein at midnight, assisted by my mother.

After most visits to our farm, he'd pop into the house with a quick hug and kiss, followed by a hurried exchange, then off to the next call as fast as he entered. It was rare for

Doc to take a break, or sit down. As one of four girls born to a busy dairy farmer and farm wife, I can relate to this lifestyle, and also to Stan's daughters who were similarly involved in a family business with the farm as its base.

Like Doc, my father enjoyed playing basketball, but never really had any "hobbies," so it was exciting and a little foreign to us when he finally traded with Stan some Holstein heifers for a pair of Belgian foals—Bud and Ben, who became known as "The Boys." Doc recalled, "Bernie came down 10 times, I'll bet, to look at those colts before he made up his mind to trade."

My dad enjoyed working with draft horses as a boy and remembered walking behind his father and their team as they raked hay. He told us how he fell asleep on the grassy knoll where my house is built today.

Also like Stan, Dad was greatly influenced by his own father, who died when he was young; and in the same fashion, my father bought the farm from his mother and siblings. To my dad, who would often start his sentences with, "When my father was alive…" it defined an era. Stan would become one of my father's mentors, and Dad would stop to visit him when things weighed on his mind. When my dad passed away a few years ago, Stan was the first of our extended family to come through my back door with a comforting hug and a knowing silence.

Although this book is dedicated to Stan and Shirley's three daughters, it is also a tribute from a daughter to my father, Bernie Palmer. One of his greatest joys was to share his own childhood stories of family and the farm. I wish I had written them down… "when my father was alive."

About the author:

Penny Heritage was one of four daughters raised on Palmer's Acres View Farm, her family's dairy farm of 345 acres, in the towns of Ballston and Charlton, in Saratoga County, New York. A graduate of Burnt Hills-Ballston Lake High School, she earned an A.A.S. in Agricultural Science from S.U.N.Y. Cobleskill, and a B.S. in Dairy Science, with concentrations in Communication Arts from Cornell University. Following an 18-year career in communications, public relations and marketing, with two organizations in the public and private sectors, Heritage followed her heart in the tradition of her agricultural roots, and made the satisfying leap to self-employment.

She contracts with the New York State Agricultural Society, and LEAD New York—the Empire State Food and Agricultural Leadership Institute, and has contributed to the New York Farmer and Country Folks newspapers. Heritage also operates her small business, Heritage Farm Originals, creating and painting agricultural designs for farms, organizations and events. Her work has been commissioned by the New York State Farm Bureau, among others, and has celebrated agriculture at legislative receptions, fairs, maple open houses, rural-urban events, educational tours, and on Christmas cards.

Burnt Hills Veterinary Tails is her first book to be produced by Heritage Farm Publishing. The author lives in the town of Charlton with her husband, Marshall, their daughter, Emma, and cat, Kiddles.

Special thanks!

Editing and Back Cover Copy
By Carrie M. Majer

Cover Design & Composition
By Tammy T. Johnson

Illustration
By Mary E. Maguire

and to Penny from Doc:

Family and friends have said for years that I should write a book. Shirley and I would start to gather information together and then get discouraged.

Penny Heritage came into the picture, enthusiastically exclaiming that she would love to help. We were at a family gathering, and as Penny's parents were dairy farm clients of mine for many years (as well as being relatives and friends) Penny had the perfect background of knowledge to put the book together.

What a great adventure it has been! Working with Penny has been lots of fun and hard work, but Shirley and I want to thank her so much and tell her how grateful we are for this book she has compiled and written. It is through her expertise, persistence, and long hours of work that it has become a reality.

Thank you, Penny, for all your help and most of all for your sunny and cheerful personality.

Order Form

Heritage Farm Publishing
493 Charlton Road
Ballston Spa, NY 12020-3203

Please send _____ copies of:

"Burnt Hills Veterinary Tails" to:

Name:_____

Address:_____

City: _____ State _____

Zip _____

Price: $20.00

Sales Tax:
New York State orders please add $1.40 sales tax per book

Shipping/Handling:
$3.00 for the first book, $2.00 for each additional book shipped to the same address.

Please remit check or money order payable to:
Heritage Farm Publishing

Total amount enclosed: _____

Orders also online at: www.heritagefarmpublishing.com